I thought it offered a fresh, honest, clear, and direct perspective. The voice of a mother who left her comfort zone, studied the issue, did research, and started to change her eating habits, a process that she generously shares with us. At times, I heard the voice of Hygieia—the symbolical mother, wife, and daughter of Asclepius. Hygieia represents hygiene, proper diets, exercise, rest, and care. I also heard the voice of Mother Nature, who shows us the consequences that our individual and collective behaviors have on this environment that has given us a home and shelter and provided for us throughout centuries...

Dr. Marco Aurelio Macías, Surgeon and Doctor of Holistic Naturism, Former President of the Latin American Society of Natural Medicine

Healthy Planet, Healthy You *is a gift for each of us and, at the same time, a gesture of care and comprehension for this world that gives us a home and sustenance. Ximena's straightforward, friendly, and smart narrative takes us by the hand to individually contribute to a paradigm change in our eating habits and well-being.*

Lorenzo J. de Rosenzweig P., visual artist, Founder and CEO of Terra Habitus, AC, Founder of Fondo Mexicano para la Conservación de la Naturaleza, AC, Former President of the Network of Latin American and Caribbean Environmental Funds, Former President of the Board of the Mesoamerican Reef Fund

A piece full of bravery, honesty, and research that opens our eyes to the reality of our current eating habits and how they relate to the planet's health. Healthy Planet, Health You *invites us to ask questions and do research from our role as consumers and start changing paradigms so we can care for the health of our two homes: our bodies and the planet Earth. An exceptional book that we should all read.*

Dr. Marili Leopold Sordo Integrative Doctor at Dr. Weil Center for Integrative Medicine

A clear explanation of personal experiences that will be incredibly useful for those who want to experience new ways of living so they can be better inhabitants of this planet. Destroy as little as possible and coexist in a better and healthier way in the time that we are destined to share on EARTH. *A book that should be read carefully.*

Dr. María del Carmen Onega Clinical Gynecologist with a specialty in Gynecological Endocrinology and Osteoporosis and Osteopenia Treatment

At many stages of our lives, we aren't mindful and don't develop our personal resources until we take a strong hit...until we get into an accident or face a circumstance that pushes us to make significant changes. Presenting very timely information, Ximena invites us to reflect on the implications of everything from the sales of large corporations to the daily decisions we make about the food we eat. This is a call to pay attention, an invitation to gain awareness and adapt to the big changes that are approaching, which we can actively and creatively take part in.

Isabel Barraza
L&D Palliative Care, Innovation, & Design Thinking,
Experts in Change Palliative Care Consultant and Innovation Teacher

In this book, Ximena opens your eyes to a new way of living that is friendlier with the planet. She does this through a simple but brilliant proposal of caring for the environment while simultaneously improving your health. Telling us about the path she has taken and her experience of change, she recommends that we also follow it to the extent that is possible for us. Not only does she provide us with the tools for making these changes, but she also gives us the foundations. Taking us by the hand in a friendly and natural way, she makes us wonder: What are we doing to change things? Hopefully we all join in on her proposal.

Roxana Iglesias
Nutritionist and Food Scientist

HEALTHY PLANET, HEALTHY YOU

Simple Habits to Create a Brighter Future

XIMENA YÁÑEZ SOTO

*Translated from the original Spanish
by Laura Elliott*

HEALTHY PLANET, HEALTHY YOU
Simple Habits to Create a Brighter Future

ISBN: 978-1-7378678-2-1

Printed in the United States of America

To Mother Earth and to the future generations,
so they might mutually enjoy each other
for a long, long time to come.

CONTENTS

ACKNOWLEDGMENTS

I have the most sincere and profound gratitude for all those who have come along with me in this process.

I'll start with my family, Luis and my daughters Camila and Emilia, for their infinite patience over the long weekends when I buried myself in research, writing, design, editing, and corrections.

To Mariana, my sister, my confidant, my personal cheerleader, my conscience, because without her in my life, my light would not be the same.

To those who took this book on as their personal project and devoted long hours to helping me realize my dream: the extraordinary mentor and guide that life gave me, Lorenzo Rosenzweig, and my dear friend, Adrián Gutiérrez, whose unconditional support made everything possible.

To my relentless critics, my brother Bernardo, my cousin Roxana Iglesias, and also to Manuel Molano and Federico Llamas, because their candid feedback motivated me to clarify many of my ideas and go further in depth in my research.

To my content and format editors, because their comments helped me allow my ideas to flow naturally. To my father, José Manuel; Cuca Lomelín; my aunt Elvira Yáñez; Araceli Sánchez; María Isabel Barraza; Adriana Fournier; my uncle Max Alberto Soto; Jimena González; Mónica Narro; Eli García; and Oli Martínez.

To my accountability partner, Yose Pérez, for listening to me week after week and guiding me until I found my voice.

To my daughter Camila, for the beautiful illustrations that accompany each of the recipes.

To the chef who believed in this dream and created the original recipes for this book, Natalia Delgado.

To Pope Francis for encouraging me to persevere with hope in my good intentions, which he expressed in his response to a letter I sent him about this project, sent through the Apostolic Nunciature in Washington, D.C.

To Laura Elliott, for her accurate feedback and whose translation was meticulous and very well done. She totally understood where I come from and the key message I want to share.

To my beautiful friend Mary Giuseffi, for seeing my potential and offering her unconditional support to bring life to the dream of getting this message out into the world.

Thanks also to all those who enthusiastically motivated me to follow my dream when the idea for this book was merely a thought floating around inside my head.

I lack the words to describe and express all the gratitude I feel, so for just a few seconds, I'll take the famous phrase of the master Gustavo Cerati and make it mine:

A todos ustedes ¡gracias totales!
(To all of you, absolute thanks!)

WARNING:
THIS BOOK
ISN'T FOR YOU IF...

S ome say there are none so blind as those who do not want to see...

This is not a science book. In it, I speak of our current environmental situation, about the projections for the coming years, and about how our patterns of consumption are related to the deterioration of the environment and our health. While this book does compile some statistics and present some correlations between different variables—such as those between the intake of certain foods and different diseases—the bases of these associations have yet to be scientifically proven. Consequently, while these factors are obviously related, they lack the scientific support, and seemingly, for those who base all their actions on science, this is the requisite condition for making any change in their lives. Despite having devoted many years to studying the relationship between nutrition, general well-being, and holistic health, I've had occasional conversations about these issues in which my arguments have been seen as pseudoscience, conjectures, intuition, or unfounded theories.

Yet, the truth of the matter is that these topics are hard to exclusively address from science because there are many variables in the relationship between health and eating that would lose their value as a comprehensive issue if they were studied in isolation.

Moreover, studies performed on human beings cannot be done in contained and controlled environments, as with rats or other lab animals. So, when I share more abstract ideas in these kinds of discussions, it's because I think that, while science does have exact answers for an infinite number of issues, there are others whose answers are not definitive. And in no way am I saying that science is useless. Rather, my point is that for certain subjects—including nutrition—we still don't have the skills or tools to understand them, analyze them, and reach exact conclusions when we study them. Today, the science behind nutrition is a romantic idea that we can confirm without giving it much thought: a diet that is good for one person might be poison for another.

When I get into debates on these issues, I think that strictly sticking to the science can blind us (or give us a certain sense of arrogance) and make us incapable of going beyond our intellectual knowledge to use our eyes and see our reflection in a mirror. And I stress this because I've found that those who engage in these types of arguments are often ignoring their own health issues. This is why I say there are none so blind as those who do not want to see. The problem is that they're not the only ones who suffer from their health conditions—their families are also victims.

This book is not for those who cannot see beyond scientific arguments that, in excess, are just as damaging as their extreme opposite. These are the same people who treat science as another "dogma of faith," which does not allow them to accept that it is inevitably confined to the sensorial limitations of human beings. They are the same people who discredit hypotheses backed by correlations, patterns, and tendencies, even when it is apparent that something is happening that requires further study and action.

This book isn't for those who aren't open to new opportunities either, because it will be incredibly difficult for them to see the world from different perspectives… Or for those who are not willing to think outside the box because, undoubtedly, you'll find topics in this book that will push you away from traditional thought patterns.

It is not for those who have settled firmly into their comfort zones, because leaving this zone will have an impact on different aspects of your life, which can sometimes be intensely unsettling. This includes those who have found the solution for their health problems with a diet that's heavily based on animal products, because these people have already defined their priorities.

It is not for those who go about life ignoring others' pain, because it's clear that nothing will soften their hearts, or for those who have already lost hope in humanity and think small changes will never be enough.

It is not for anyone who doesn't believe that human beings are also spiritual beings or for those who evade their responsibility to the planet and to the living beings we share it with, because what I am going to share here won't make any sense to them.

Naturally, it's not for those who don't believe the words of someone who, despite having studied the issue for almost ten years, does not have an academic degree to back up those years of study.

Sadly, this book is not for people who believe that the changes to their lives and habits, which their families urgently need, can keep waiting.

If none of the above applies to you, welcome! I'd like to invite you to read this book with an open heart and mind.

INTRODUCTION

For over 20 years, I worked at an environmental fund with hopes of building a better future for my home country of Mexico, for the world, and for our children. Like many others, I thought the actions needed to stop and reverse the degradation of natural resources were the responsibility of the government and civil society organizations. I thought it was easy to bury my head in the sand or turn a blind eye by making a few environmentally responsible adjustments at home but then leaving the major conservation challenges to the big-timers: to those who are visible and have a voice.

Then, a couple of years ago, I had a dream that hit me like a pail of cold water: I dreamt my great-great-granddaughter asked me what I had done for the planet when I heard about the problems our modern lifestyle would eventually cause for future generations... With a knot in my chest and unable to answer, I realized that leaving all the work and responsibility to these major stakeholders was not enough.

In March 2019, the United Nations (UN) published its sixth Global Environment Outlook report "GEO-6: Healthy Planet, Healthy People," which states that we have bleak prospects for reaching sustainable development by 2050 and calls on us to adopt urgent measures as individuals. This document concludes that, despite the environmental policy efforts that all the governments have pursued, our anthropogenic actions (an uncommon term that means "consequences of human behavior") of production and consumption are unsustainable and also the main reason why ecosystems continue to degrade and deteriorate around the entire world.

We cannot keep waiting for others to change our planet's destiny. It's time to heed the warnings about the kind of future we are leaving for our children, to take them seriously and do everything within reach to reverse the deterioration from where we stand…

…now, while there's still time.

Perhaps you've had the same experience as I have: You get overloaded with information about the expected outlook in 20 or 30 years, but the suggestions for change are so overwhelming that you put them aside and wait for others to solve what seems impossible. Maybe you feel small or insignificant before the size of the challenge we're facing, and so you lower your head, assuming your individual actions couldn't change a thing. The good news is that there is something we can do if we work together, if we organize ourselves into an army of millions who all make a small change at the same time. With enough knowledge, you can start to make these small changes in your daily life, and, if they are replicated, they'll have an exponential effect, just like ripples in the water.

In this book, I'll talk about animal proteins: the role that our immoderate consumption of them plays in the planet's deterioration; the myths and ideologies surrounding their nutritional value, which we have grown up with and then turned into laws; and, yes, I'll also discuss the health risks we are facing because of the excesses we've reached. Likewise, I'll show you how, for years, our heads have been filled with lies that have turned into paradigms based on repetition and a lack of questioning; how the media has manipulated us; what mechanisms the food industry uses to make us addicted to the products they sell; and how, with a small change at home, we can have a positive environmental impact. I'll speak of the role human beings play in the deterioration of the environment and in animal abuse and also about our responsibilities as individuals and societies. We'll take a quick tour of the little-known world of microorganisms, which our health is largely dependent on, and we'll review some innovative research that's crucial if we are going to dare to change. We'll also go back in time briefly to learn the opinions of some philosophers and thinkers. I'll interweave personal experiences with statistics and hard facts, but I'll speak from the heart so that everything I tell you about here will be entertaining and easy to understand. Some people have asked me to include examples of how I deal with the flood of (mis)information. So, at the end of certain chapters, I'll tell you what I do, but please keep in mind that this is how I face my day-to-day life. You should make your own decisions based on what works best for you and according to your unique circumstances. When I refer to the food industry, I'll mainly be discussing animal products, and I'll use statistics from the United States because it's the global benchmark and, generally speaking, its practices permeate the rest of the world.

My intention is that we do this together, step by step. I want to help you remove the veils that others have covered your eyes with and equip you with the tools you'll need to gain awareness about the world that surrounds us and understand the long-term effects of our actions. Over the course of this book, I'll tell you about the environmental and health implications of our current eating patterns to encourage you to make a small change in your lifestyle that will, undoubtedly, contribute to the process of transformation that the world needs. Don't worry, you don't have to feel like you're carrying the weight of the world on your shoulders. We're on this ride together.

Also, I should warn you that this book is like a Pandora's box: If you close it right now, you'll go back to life as you know it, and nothing will have happened that could put your world off-kilter. If you decide to keep reading, you'll see that some of the things you took for granted for a long time are not what they seemed to be, which will drive you to see the world with new eyes. I intend to explain what's going on in the world from another perspective, and if you decide to embark on this adventure with me, we'll travel together to the greatest depths of the rabbit hole. So, if you're sticking with me, I recommend that you fasten your seat belt because, as Cypher told Neo in the movie *The Matrix* when alluding to Dorothy's trip in the *Wizard of Oz*, "Kansas is going bye-bye…"[1]

---

[1] *The Matrix*, 1999.

✌ 1 ✎

A BIT ABOUT ME

WHERE I COME FROM AND WHERE I'M GOING

There wasn't hype or fanfare. On my last day of work, I signed the corresponding paperwork and, with my emotions running high, I wrote a goodbye letter to all those with whom I had formed some type of relationship during my time at the organization. I received a marginal response to that letter, and feeling somewhat hurt and deeply saddened, I confirmed what we all know but that's hard to accept: no one is indispensable. That was how, from a place in my soul, I forced an end to what had been my professional project for over 23 years.

An important part of my job was overseeing control and compliance for a Mexican environmental fund that channels financial resources toward protecting the country's natural wealth. Five years earlier, my family and I had left Mexico to follow my husband's professional dreams and, since my work consisted of meeting requirements and safeguarding the institution's interests, it was always quite clear to me that the day would come when the board of directors would have to replace me. Plus, my family responsibilities were growing, which meant the time available to me for working had become very limited. For five years, I tried to prepare myself mentally and emotionally, but when the fund's directors decided it was time to look for someone new, my heart sank into a whirlwind of emotions. On the one hand, I felt a huge relief because I knew that, if I were to continue this long-distance work, the stress of not having enough time would start to affect my health. On the other hand, I also knew my dreams of retiring from this institution—which I'd helped build with so much love and that I was so grateful for—were over.

It was time to start looking for what I would do once I disengaged from the professional life that had driven me for so many years.

One day, while browsing Facebook, I came across an ad for a health coach training at an integrative nutrition institute. Several years earlier, I'd discovered that my health (which had been deteriorating for many years) improved significantly when I made some changes to my lifestyle and began to understand the relationship between diet and well-being. I was drawn to the idea of learning how to help other people achieve what I had believed impossible at a certain stage of my life: enjoying good health. This institute was offering me a truly comprehensive training program aimed at exploring and understanding different sources of nutrition for human beings: from the tangible aspects of nutrition based on bio-individuality to concepts of primary foods, which include, among others, spirituality, professional development, personal relationships, recreation, rest, and physical exercise. Now, I really would have the necessary tools to inspire and help others find balance and integrative health.

So, I decided to turn over a new page in my life and embark on this journey to gain the knowledge that would enable me to help others. I had to make a 180-degree turn and relearn the basics of human relationships. I have to admit that my working experience had desensitized me from understanding the needs of others, which is why, for many years, I had been labeled an insensitive, uncompromising, and harsh person. The Mexican tax system is complicated enough as it is (those who pay taxes in Mexico know I'm not lying), but its regulations for non-profit organizations include a number of additional twists, turns, angles, and varied legal interpretations. Ensuring impeccable compliance became my professional goal. There wasn't room to include people in my world, and, indeed, I left very little maneuvering space to consider and understand that each case is special. In good nature (and obviously behind my back), my colleagues nicknamed me "Dr. No."

The good thing is that when I studied to become an integrative nutritional health coach, I had to relearn how to listen with my heart and take off the armor that I'd been building around it for years to protect my emotions. So, when I finished studying, I was ready to ask myself the mandatory question: How do I link my work in environmental conservation with this new professional adventure in which feeling and helping people have become my life's purpose? After twenty-three years in the field of conservation and almost ten years studying different schools of thought in the world of nutrition and integrative health, I've been able to untangle some of the reasons why we continue repeating patterns that turn out to be self-destructive.

As a civil organization, the fund is a global example of success because it has known how to work together with the government, institutions, civil society, and grassroots groups. Likewise, it has touched the hearts of many communities (especially indigenous and marginalized communities) that have returned to their roots: working for and with the Earth. Yet, the work of institutions like the fund is still not enough if we consider the speed at which our habits and consumption patterns continue to deteriorate the world. We have to make a change from the core of society, because neither governments nor companies are going to take the first step. That's how I got the idea to write this book and tell you an important part of the story of our planet's erosion and how it's interwoven with our waning health and quality of life.

I'll start by telling you my own story about animal protein, but in no way will I ask you to make it yours. We are all unique and unrepeatable, and the diet and lifestyle that work for one person might not be the best option for someone else. The story about what you decide to eat is yours, and I would never try to suggest that mine is better: mine is better for me, you'll decide what is better for you. All I want to do is demystify some beliefs that have been branded on the collective unconscious and made into laws that no one dares to question, and then I'll show you how we have been manipulated for the financial benefit of a few.

Hopefully this book helps you dispel the confusion backed by the food industry, which has led us to lose touch with the planet and the creatures that share it with us. This is the same industry that has strived to make us believe we are independent from our surroundings and that the only way to be happy is by consuming excessively and hoarding the resources our planet provides for us.

My wish is to show you that the planet's health and the common welfare have never gone separate ways. The illusory separation and the damage it has entailed are simply the result of our contemporary way of life, driven by egocentric economic models that have been imposed upon us. We have a lot to do, but don't despair— every journey starts with the first step.

I'D LIKE A TACO WITH EVERYTHING...EXCEPT MEAT!

"Where do you get your protein from?" This is the question that anyone who has stopped eating animal products expects to hear before responding, maybe even pretty tastelessly, with an answer that's an inside joke for those of us who follow a plant-based diet.

I stopped eating animal products a number of years ago. I didn't do it for my health or out of conviction. I simply felt the universe—or life—was trying to send me a sign, because everything I read, saw, or talked about in conversations always led me to the same conclusion. So, I decided to pay attention to this (not so hidden) message, and I stopped eating animal products. I admit that I felt somewhat afraid, because I didn't have any information that guaranteed I would continue to obtain the nutrients I needed to stay healthy. I also couldn't keep ignoring the signs from the universe that were popping up everywhere, however.

And so, full of uncertainty, I began this journey on my own. At home, I continued making "normal" food for my family, and I explored with something free of animal protein for me. The idea was to start with a trial and discovery phase in my own body. If this diet had any deficiencies, I didn't want my family to suffer the consequences.

Then, I joined a few social media groups to understand a little more about this world that was so unknown and distant to me. First, I found a group named "Veganism 101," which I ran away from a few months later when I realized that being vegan was not the same as eating a healthy diet. Veganism refers to the practice of not ingesting or using any type of product of animal origin, whether it's from the animal itself or a by-product (like eggs or cheese), products that animals produce (like honey), items derived from animals (like hides and leather), or products tested on animals (like cosmetics). However, it's perfectly possible for a vegan diet to consist of chips, cookies, high-fructose corn syrup, and soft drinks, because its only intention is to protect animals.

Another school of thought that prescribes avoiding the intake of meat but does include eggs, cheese, and honey is known as vegetarianism. Generally speaking, the base of a meal in these two practices is formed by large amounts of processed grains like bread, pasta, and boxed cereal. Some vegetarians do include fish in their diets, and this modality is known as semi-vegetarianism or pescetarianism. In short, there are different tendencies with varied interests, beliefs, and aims. I lean toward what is known as WFPBD. (No, it's not a swear word but rather the abbreviation for "whole food plant-based diet.") That's why—after leaving the Veganism 101 group—I decided to join a group with these characteristics. I must confess that I also avoid gluten as much as possible. (Yes, when I go to a restaurant, the waiter's best recommendation is to call a cab…)

At this time, I had already begun studying to be an integrative nutritional coach, and some of the seminars were taught by doctors who endorsed diets with low or zero content from animal products. (I'll admit that there were others who suggested the exact opposite.) Yet, listening to the arguments from the doctors who recommended reducing or limiting animal products from our diets, my uncertainty started to fade and give way to such vivid clarity that I was amazed I hadn't seen it years earlier.

"Where do you get your protein from?"…Finally, I heard the long-awaited question from someone very close to me, whom I love very much. With my chest puffed out and my voice charged with passion, I answered with the argument I had been preparing in my head for months: "From the same place that your proteins get their proteins."

I remember how she looked at me with big eyes and a loving smile, and, puffing out my chest even further to the sound of an imaginary fanfare, how I thought I'd given her one of those "aha-moments." Maybe just because she loves me so much and is very patient with me, she kept a warm expression on her face and, in an affectionate tone, asked, "And what does that mean?" Right then, my chest deflated, the imaginary fanfare was interrupted by the wheeze of an out-of-tune flute, and my voice cut out. Who did I think I was to give such an arrogant reply? This answer does not welcome dialogue, and, undoubtedly, its intention is to make the other person feel bad. The right response is to take my conversation partner by the hand and be patient, just as time had led me along patiently for all these years.

If you were wondering about this same question and the answer also left you totally confused, don't worry. This book is not meant to convert you to veganism or make you go WFPBD (no cursing intended). I assure you that you'll continue to make your own decisions about what you eat, but you'll be more informed when you make those decisions. My intention is to offer you the clarity that I discovered on my personal exploration so you can analyze it with your unique and special eyes and, if you think it's interesting, you can share this knowledge with your family, friends, and community—but especially with your children. Remember, it's their quality of life that's at stake.

THE THIEF WHO LEFT BEHIND THE MOON

There's a Zen tale about a wise man who lived very happily in a cabin in the mountains. He spent his days writing poetry, practicing calligraphy, playing with the town children, and helping the poor in the community.

One afternoon, while he was attending to a few matters in town, a thief broke into his home. The thief looked for something to steal, but the poet had nothing more than a paintbrush, paper, and food for his dinner.

On his way home, the wise man ran into the thief as he was about to flee. The sage stopped him and said, "Thank you for taking the time to come visit me. You must have come a long way and perhaps you're tired. Don't leave empty-handed. Please, take my clothes, as a gift."

Taken aback, the thief accepted the clothes and slipped through the darkness without saying a word.

With peace in his heart, the poet sat and stared at the night sky. "Poor man," he sighed. "I would have liked to have given him this beautiful moon!"

Then he took his paintbrush and a paper and wrote:

"The thief left behind
the moon
in my window..."

In all cultures, civilizations, societies, and religions, there are precepts and norms that serve as a basis to govern the social and moral conducts of every group. There are norms of coexistence that are exclusive to each culture, but then there are others of a more general nature. "Do not steal" is one of these universal rules that every society punishes in its own way. The punishments cover a wide range from judicial processes, fines, and social rejection to prison, stoning, and flogging, and, in the most unforgiving societies, amputations or the death penalty. There are other societies in which stealing is certainly considered a crime, but there is so much robbery—on so many different levels and with such scant punishment—that we learn to live by protecting ourselves from others.

When we are victims of robbery, we look for ways to demand justice because it's offensive to us to feel stripped of what is legitimately ours. Many of us respect what doesn't belong to us, just as we would like others to respect what does belong to us. Our conscience is at peace because we know we haven't stolen from anyone, but how true is this belief of ours?

The definition of stealing that I like the most is one I heard in a lecture from a Buddhist master: "Stealing is taking something that has not been freely given to us." This means that we also steal when we borrow something and don't return it or when we don't pay the price that something is actually worth. But there are other ways to steal: we steal someone's word when we interrupt their story to tell ours, even if we are doing it as a show of solidarity and empathy; we can also steal someone's time when we make them wait; we steal trust from others when we repeat a secret that wasn't ours to tell; we steal from the company where we work when we waste time or spend it doing things for our personal lives; and we steal from ourselves when we do things that cause us harm (and knowing this ahead of time), such as smoking, drinking excessively, or eating foods that are not good for our health. So, we can steal more than just material goods: we can also steal the future.

The future does not belong to you, or me, or anyone. It's something that does not exist now, but it is highly dependent on what we do at this time. My actions can transform into a future full of life or into a devastating scenario. If my actions of today will result in the deterioration of conditions in the future, then I am stealing from the planet and from future generations. "Twenty percent of the world's population consumes resources at a rate that robs the poor nations and future generations of what they need to survive."[2]

Like the wise man from the story, Earth gives us all it has. She provides us a home and sustenance, and she even gives us the gift of a beautiful view of the moon. We are the thieves who, without knowing why and without saying a word, slip away into the night with our booty. We probably don't realize it, but our current lifestyles are leaving a trail of destruction behind each and every one of our steps. The irony of this is that the footprint of deterioration that we shape with our excessive exploitation and production systems will only be to our own detriment as human beings. We know the Earth will recover from our selfish, egocentric practices, but if we continue at the pace of the erosion we have provoked, it's probable that this healing process will not include us as a species and, sadly, the future generations will be the ones who suffer the consequences. The actions we take today steal quality of life away from the futures of our children, our grandchildren, and of the generations to follow.

The purpose of this book is to invite you to gain awareness of what you are putting on your plate and the reasons why what seems like a trivial and harmless decision is affecting your surroundings. I'll also offer you some tips and suggestions that can be of help in case you decide to join the process of change that—if fortunate enough to

---

[2] Encyclical letter *Laudato Si'* of the Holy Father Francis on the care of our common home.

be replicated among your family, friends, and community—will be a new light of hope for the future. Yet, to have the capacity to make this change, you should revisit the relationship our ancestors had with food and the land that provided it for them: a relationship of service and respect for nature and its fruits. You can start by doing the conscious exercise of asking yourself where the meals you put on the table come from and what their environmental impact was. If you don't know or if you are not sure, perhaps it's better for you to avoid it and, instead, offer yourself and your loved ones food that has been grown or produced in harmony with the planet. By creating this awareness, you will reclaim the bond with the Earth that makes you part of her and her part of you. Let yourself be surprised by what she has to offer you, because her resources belong to you. Don't forget, though, that they also belong to those with whom you are obligated to share. But then what can we do to stop stealing from the future?

The actions you take today can be part of the deterioration or part of the change to save the planet: it's your call. However, if you decide that your actions of today are the change the planet needs, you will be giving a better future to the generations to come. A small change in your lifestyle is the first step toward discovering the satisfaction of living in harmony with the world around you. There is no greater joy than being part of the solution, and there is no greater tranquility for the soul than knowing you are a reformed thief. So, with peace in your heart, you'll feel inspired to sit and ponder the moon that the poet left for you in the window, awaiting the day when you can truly see it with new eyes…

✌ 2 ✍

WHAT'S GOING ON WITH THE WORLD?

THE HAND THAT ROCKS THE CRADLE

There's this relative of mine who sometimes makes me laugh and, other times, makes me cry... He's as stubborn as a mule and likes to believe that the way he perceives and interprets the world is the "absolute truth." He lives on a warm beach in a tropical country, sleeps in a hammock hung between two palm trees, and spends his days fully entertained with dancing, laughter, drinks, parties, and a search to prove that conspiracy theories are real. This is how he experiences his day-to-day life, and this is the information he receives directly from the world around him. With such a relaxed lifestyle, he's very active on social media, and he loves to argue...surely because he enjoys creating controversies and getting into never-ending pointless debates. If most of his social media contacts are in favor of something, he immediately looks for some contradictory publication or study and posts it without missing a beat.

This is an example of how, even if we live in a fantasy land that's completely isolated from the rest of the world, we have the means to receive information in real time. The problem is that information has become excessively confusing, because we might quickly find a study that reaches one conclusion, but then we instantly find another that contradicts it. The amount and diversity of information we're exposed to keeps us on a rollercoaster of hard facts, statements, and contradictions: what was good a few years ago isn't anymore and vice versa; the trends change from one minute to the next. In order to sort through this sea of information and decide what to pay attention to according to the best of your knowledge and understanding, my advice is that you find out where the studies are getting their funding from—that is, "follow the money."

Sadly, when speaking of nutrition and health, some institutions—whose main purpose is to protect us as a society and as human beings—would *seem* to be neutral sources, but the truth is that many private entities (like the food and pharmaceutical industries) invest large amounts of financial resources in them. For example, if a study that catches your eye is government sponsored, consider that the government receives large sums of money through lobbying, financial support for political campaigns, subsidies for social causes the government does not have the capacity to manage, gifts, the funding of political events, and practices such as "check-offs" and "revolving doors."

The "revolving door" is the common practice of 1) hiring former public officials to hold key positions in lobbying groups and 2) nominating former directors of lobbying groups for government positions. Moreover, "check-offs" are a tax deduction for earnings from food products sales. In an ideal world, the government would first invest in research and then in general advertising expenses. Unfortunately, the funds raised through check-offs are invested less in research and more in advertising campaigns that specifically promote the same products that generated the money to begin with. The top examples of this type of practice are the campaigns that promote milk and dairy products as the best source of calcium as well as those that claim the cholesterol in eggs is healthy and that lean meat is good for your heart.

I would like to consider universities, think tanks, and private associations as neutral sources, but what is actually going on is that many faculties and departments are also subsidized and funded by both the food industry and the pharmaceutical industry, or "big pharma." I'll give you some examples: In 1998, the University of California Berkeley (UC Berkeley) signed a partnership agreement with the Swiss agricultural and pharmaceutical company Novartis, which also owns Gerber products. For Berkeley, this partnership represented a capital input of $50 million over a 5-year period (half of this money would be allocated to laboratories and the other half to funding studies). At the time, this figure was a third of the Department of Agricultural & Resource Economics' total annual budget. Debates surrounding these types of practices focus on whether or not academic institutions are truly independent and autonomous from their financial sponsors.

Here are some other examples of private associations that receive industry funding: 1) The American Council on Science and Health (ACSH), which is a non-profit group whose representatives frequently discuss food issues, basing their comments on the results of scientific studies. Although it keeps its corporate donor list private, the consumer advocacy organization Center for Science in the Public Interest (CSPI) detected that at least 40% of this association's funding comes from the food industry, especially from meat and cooking oil products. 2) The American Heart Association (AHA), which raises funds through membership dues. In this case, the products of the companies that are part of the program—and pay the corresponding dues—receive the "heart-healthy" label. 3) American Dietetic Association (ADA), which is a professional association that represents the interests of a group of associate nutrition professionals (registered dietitians). Many of its members are employed by the food industry, and the ADA also receives donations from this same industry. Its members base their recommendations on brands, arguing that there are no good or bad foods.

In addition to the sponsorship money that research centers and universities receive from the industry, there is a common practice of sharing staff. This situation has been seriously questioned and exposed as a conflict of interests. If you want to learn the details about how relationships between the industry and the government, think tanks, and nutrition professional associations are managed, I recommend you read the book *Food Politics: How the Food Industry Influences Nutrition and Health* by Dr. Marion Nestle.

We also face the limitation of what is considered a valid scientific study and, therefore, the source that governments and their respective agencies use to issue their recommendations to the population. Let me give you an example: Today, you can find varied results about the toxicity of a substance called glyphosate. Some studies conclude that it has a moderate toxicity level, while others have determined that the substance has a possible carcinogenic effect on humans. So, which ones do we believe? Glyphosate is the active substance in the herbicide that is most widely used worldwide—it's called Roundup and it's used to kill competing plants in intensive commercial farming. This herbicide does not kill the primary crop (corn, soy, cotton, canola, beets, sugarcane, alfalfa, and tobacco, among others) because the plants have been genetically modified (they are what we know as genetically modified organisms or GMOs). In broad terms, the gene of a bacterium called *Agrobacterium* sp. strain CP4, which is resistant to the herbicide, is inserted into the genetic code of these plants, and this is why the primary crop does not die when sprayed. However, the resistant plant absorbs the chemical compound, and when we eat it, we take in a considerable amount of the glyphosate that has soaked into its tissues.

Now, according to the recommendations of both governments and government agencies—such as the Environmental Protection Agency (EPA), the World Health Organization (WHO), the Food and Agriculture Organization (FAO), and the European Union (EU) —glyphosate is moderately toxic and safe for mammals, but there must be a warning label. However, in 2015, the International Agency for Research on Cancer (IARC) presented a study on glyphosate's possible carcinogenic effect on human beings. The agencies which state that glyphosate is moderately toxic based their conclusions on "formal" studies done on mice and rats but conducted and funded by the industry. In contrast, the IARC based its conclusions on health monitoring of farmers and consumers who were exposed to the substance. Unfortunately, since the latter was not carried out in a lab (which would have made it possible to isolate the variables and components), it is not replicable and, therefore, is a study "without scientific basis." Consequently, since the industry-subsidized studies are "replicable," they are still considered scientifically valid for determining this chemical compound's toxicity levels regardless of the individual experiences of the thousands of people whom this substance has affected.

My brother, who's a scientist, says that researchers are very vigilant about their research processes and that, sooner or later, (clarifying that it's not immediate because science takes time) the biased studies are brought out into the open, and the scientists who were involved lose their credibility. The problem with health and food related research results is that we don't have the luxury of waiting. Because waiting for the truth to fall of its own weight was what allowed the tobacco industry to present scientific studies for years that hid the harmful effects of smoking. This confusion, created by manipulated studies, even led medical journals to include advertising that targeted smokers. It is true that honest science prevailed, and the necessary measures were taken to inform consumers about the harm smoking can cause. The problem is that it took over forty years (the disputes started in 1964), and during this time, the industry continued to generate earnings estimated at $280 billion. Many people whose health and quality of life were directly and indirectly affected by cigarettes had to wait years for the truth to come out.

Honestly, I think we deserve better as a society. (Or could it be that we already have what we deserve?)

Currently, the soft drink and sugar industries have funded hundreds of scientific studies that conclude that consuming soft drinks, sugar, and artificial sweeteners has no health repercussions. Specifically, between 2010 and 2015, Coca-Cola invested more than $120 million in universities and think tanks with the aim of funding research on the issue of overweight and obesity. Likewise, according to a study published by Cambridge University Press in March 2018,[3] from 2008 to 2016, it backed 389 articles published in 169 journals that conclude exercise is key to losing weight and consuming soft drinks does not play a role in this important health issue.[4] The journal *Annals of Internal Medicine* published an article in August 2017 that determines there is not enough evidence to support the relationship between sugar consumption and negative health effects, which is why our diets should not place limits on sugar intake.[5] What's interesting about this study is that it was backed by the Life Science Institute, a group funded by Coca-Cola and whose sponsors include, among others, Bayer, DuPont, General Mills, Hershey Foods, Kellogg's,

[3] Serôdio, PM, et al. "Coca-Cola – A Model of Transparency in Research Partnerships? A Network Analysis of Coca-Cola's Research Funding (2008–2016)." *Public Health Nutr.* 2018 Jun.
[4] Hyman, Mark, *Food Fix: How to Save Our Health, Our Economy, Our Communities, and Our Planet – One Bite at a Time.* 180.
[5] Yeung, C. Albert, "The Scientific Basis of Guideline Recommendations on Sugar Intake." *Annals of Internal Medicine.* August, 2017.

Kraft, McDonald's, Monsanto, Nestle, Novartis, PepsiCo, Pfizer, and Procter & Gamble.[6]

Another example is ketchup, which is cataloged as a "healthy food" under the argument that, despite being a highly processed food loaded with sugar and salt (1 tablespoon = 4 grams of added sugar and 190 milligrams of sodium), it contains high levels of the antioxidant lycopene, which is naturally found in tomatoes. The argument is supported by a study conducted in 2004 by the Harvard School of Public Health, which revealed that women with high levels of lycopene in their blood have a lower risk (50%) of developing coronary diseases.

Also relating to processed tomatoes, there's an interesting story behind why tomato paste receives special treatment in school lunch regulation in the United States. According to the guidelines, ⅛ cup of tomato puree has the same nutritional value as ½ cup of vegetables. So, it's not that school boards think a slice of pizza is a vegetable, but because it has tomato paste, it's given the same nutritional value as a cup of vegetables. And the main issue is that this type of information confuses consumers because it makes them think that including ketchup or pizza in their diets is good for their health.

As Dr. Mark Hyman would say, the food industry manages society, public opinion, the government, and, quite unfortunately, science. (In the United States, the government invests approximately $1 billion each year in nutrition research, while the food industry invests an annual $12 billion.) The result? Confusion among doctors, nutritionists, society, and those who develop public policies. In his book, *Food Fix: How to Save Our Health, Our Economy, Our Communities, and Our Planet—One Bite at a Time,* Dr. Hyman presents information verifying that studies funded by the industry reach conclusions in its own benefit 8 to 50 times more than independently conducted

---

[6] Hyman, Mark, *Food Fix: How to Save Our Health, Our Economy, Our Communities, and Our Planet – One Bite at a Time.*

studies, and he ends by asserting that nutrition science is heavily corrupted. For example, a 2017 analysis published in the *Journal of the American Medical Association* (JAMA) determined that, compared to independent studies, those funded by the industry are 30% more likely to reach conclusions favoring their sponsors. Another example is that, despite their high fat and sugar content, more than 50 products developed by Kellogg's—including boxed cereals such as Froot Loops and Trix—have the AHA's "heart-healthy" label. Isn't it interesting that similar products developed by other companies that don't pay membership dues are excluded from these labels?

Following the same line, in his book *The China Study: Startling Implications for Diet, Weight Loss and Long-Term Health,* Dr. T. Colin Campbell narrates a series of personal experiences tied to using the results of cancer-related research inappropriately. These experiences reveal the dark side of science and formal research: the manipulation and misuse of information that take place behind the scenes in matters of health and food policy-making. These abuses of power do not harm only honest scientists and researchers who cross paths with large industries, but, along the way, they affect the entire society.

In no way am I trying to say that I'm against science, and I completely agree with what my brother says: "Science is a systematic way of carefully observing and understanding nature and of consistently using logic to evaluate results." And, certainly, we need explanations for principles and causes as well as the formulation and testing of hypotheses. I believe that science is a true gift from and for humanity when it is used impartially for the common benefit. The problem isn't science itself—the problem is the way the empowered food industry misuses scientific studies for its own benefit. As my husband's grandad would very elegantly say, *"poderoso caballero es don Dinero"* (which translates to something like "Mr. Money is a powerful gentleman").

It's clear that the food industry's main goal is to sell us their products, sometimes at any cost. So, we should be careful and question the soundness of their arguments. Remember, when we ask questions, we build a more solid foundation for reaching our own conclusions and making decisions to meet our specific needs better. I can imagine that the needs of my relative, the one who sleeps in a hammock in the tropics, include creating polemics and opening spaces for debate. So, he's sure to make his decisions based on the need to encourage controversial arguments. However, if your interests are related to your health, your family's health, and the planet's health, then you have to be more cautious, and you definitely must question the industry's arguments when it uses publicity stunts to ask you to consume excessive quantities of the products they sell.

What I want to make clear is that I'll never ask you to blindly believe what I share here. What I'm presenting is not the result of my own scientific research and much less of my erudition or of a spontaneous flash of illumination. It comes from many years of tasking myself with reviewing and studying varied research on matters of health, nutrition, and eating that was, indeed, conducted by scientists. It's the result of making decisions about how I would relate to food when I was finding conclusions that were diametrically opposite. Therefore, whenever you have questions about the validity of a study and its conclusions, I invite you to ask the question: Where did the resources to fund this study come from and who is benefiting most from the results? It's a good practice to review the formulation and testing of the hypothesis and the methods used. Yet, because of the moves large corporations make in pursuit of their interests, nowadays, it is also necessary to look into who funds the information sources that you consider to be reliable. Remember, sometimes it takes work to detect whose hand is actually rocking the cradle.

TIP #1: What can you do?

✓ To navigate your exposure to mass marketing and dishonest advertising, learn to ignore captions or labels ensuring that one product or another is good for your health, the heart, improving digestive problems, lowering cholesterol, or that it will promise to cover your daily nutritional needs. These labels and statements in favor of your health only have one objective: to sell more products.

✓ When you go to the grocery store, start with fruits and vegetables, which, paradoxically, are the products that don't need labels or marketing strategies to glorify their benefits. Fill your home with the color and energy of these products.

✓ Fruits and vegetables come in the packaging that nature provided, and when we make them a central part of our diet, we contribute to reducing the amount of trash we produce. As much as possible, avoid packaged fruits and vegetables.

✓ You'll win three times over when you increase your consumption of fruits and vegetables: 1) You won't let the industry seduce you. 2) Your health will benefit. 3) You'll contribute to lessening the serious problem of garbage production.

✓ Check that processed and packaged foods are free of transgenics and made with organic ingredients. It's important that you're aware that they are processed products, and that just because they are labeled "organic" does not mean they are healthy.

✓ Read the nutrition labels. (Careful: This information is listed according to portions and not for the total content of the package.) Check the amount of added sugar. (The daily recommendation is a maximum of six tablespoons, which equals 24 grams of sugar.) Check the types of fats. (Avoid products with saturated and trans fats as well as those made with canola or "vegetable" oil.) Finally, analyze the ingredients. If you don't know the meaning of any of the listed words, you'd be better off setting that product aside.

✓ Look for products with the fewest ingredients and know—and also understand—what each of those ingredients is.

✓ Do your research and then make your own decisions.

EXPIRATION DATE: 2050

In this chapter, I present some of the conclusions from the UN report published in March 2019. I had to do some detective work because the information was scattered…a little here and there, and a bit more over there, and then some more over there. Surely, the UN doesn't want to unleash the fury of the food industry (just wait until you read more about this in the coming chapters), and that's why it incorporated little fragments of information that are strewn throughout the entire report. You won't find what I've written here presented in the document in the same way, but if you're interested, I invite you to read the complete report and come to your own conclusions.[7]

In March 2019, the UN published the sixth "Global Environment Outlook" (GEO 6) report, which centers on the topic "healthy planet, healthy people." This report gathers the results of a series of reviews and measurements based on current environmental policies alongside a timeline of environmental conditions. Its aim is to determine the viability of sustainable development in 2050. The report closes with the unfortunate news that, despite all the efforts made surrounding environmental issues, the general state of the environment has followed a global trend toward deterioration and—even though economic development has improved access to wealth, health, and education—it will not be sustainable by 2050 if we do not make urgent changes. According to this report, our current patterns of production and consumption are unsustainable, and anthropogenic activities (those we do as human beings) have degraded all the ecosystems worldwide. The conclusion is that we should adopt "urgent measures on an unprecedented scale" to reverse

---

[7] https://www.unenvironment.org/resources/global-environment-outlook-6

these tendencies, restore the health of the environment, and guarantee human health.

The UN also puts forth that, in response to growing and changing consumer demands, the food system is heightening pressure on local and global ecosystems, and this increases the problem of climate change around the world. Our practices of exploiting natural resources put pressure on the environment and, as years go by and the population grows, they will become food sustainability challenges. By July 2021, the world population is getting closer to 7.9 billion people, and it's estimated to reach 10 billion by 2050. To feed that many people, current food production would need to increase by 50%; however, there is not enough land or water to meet this future demand. But how do our eating patterns affect the planet? The answer is that agricultural systems are inefficient and unsustainable, and they have caused a large part of the environmental degradation and loss of biological diversity because they exert the following critical pressures:

1) Soil Degradation

Agriculture is the largest anthropogenic use of land, as it covers 50% of all inhabitable terrain. The use of 77% of these crops is allocated to pastures, grasslands for ranching activities, and producing feed for farm animals. Therefore, the claim that meat products require more land than agriculture is true, since over two-thirds of all crops are used for feeding industrial farm animals.

2) Climate Change

In addition to the fossil fuels extracted and used by the industry to cover its production and transportation needs, land use and changes to landscapes, intensive cattle and farm animal breeding, agriculture, and forestry[8] are factors that cause the atmospheric concentrations of

---

[8] The science or practice of planting, managing, and caring for forests.

greenhouse gases to increase. If the current levels of greenhouse gas emissions persist, the average global temperature will continue to rise, and—between 2030 and 2050—it will exceed the mark agreed upon as part of the Paris Agreement, which is to keep global temperature rise below 2 degrees centigrade and continue efforts to limit it to 1.5 degrees centigrade.

3) Water Scarcity

Globally, agriculture is the largest consumer of water, which is why it is necessary to manage it sustainably. On average, agriculture uses 70% of freshwater resources, but in the poorest countries, this figure can be as high as 90%. Also, water quality has grown significantly worse since 1990 due to organic and chemical pollution caused by the intensive use of pesticides, herbicides, nitrogen-based fertilizers, antibiotics, hormones, and other chemical compounds such as phosphorus and arsenic that are distributed through freshwater systems in all continents as a result of agriculture, aquaculture, and the intensive breeding of cattle and other farm animals.

4) Loss of Biological Diversity

Biological diversity is key for keeping the planet's different ecosystems in balance because it regulates the climate, offers ways to filter air and water, allows healthy soil to develop, and mitigates the effects of natural phenomena. However, exhaustive food production causes the transformation, loss, and degradation of habitats; involves unsustainable agricultural practices; promotes the spread of invasive species; and requires the overexploitation of resources, such as illegal logging. This triggers a significant process of species extinction that puts the planet's integrity and its capacity to satisfy future human needs in danger.

In theory, the aim of our current economic system is to benefit the population by allocating resources through market mechanisms. This economic system, which should offer equal opportunities for all, is actually managed by large corporations that, with their slogan of "profit and progress," create inequality and encourage unsustainable exploitation, production, and consumption schemes. Certainly, wealth is a legitimate goal in all of our lives, but, as we've seen, wealth at others' expense is a form of stealing. And what's going on is that this economic system, which is inevitably replicated in our way of living, strongly impacts the rest of the world. Economic development plans have left elements like pollution, the degradation of natural systems, and other serious environmental and social pressures out of the equation. It's time to make a transformative change…

One approach to sustainable development that is actually in our hands is making a conscious shift in our mindset because, as a society, we have the power to mediate government and industry decisions. As citizens, we should demand that authorities and companies implement sustainable agricultural practices and that they integrate concepts of environmental circularity. We should also move toward a sustainable diet that creates synergy between our health and the planet's health to contribute to reducing the loss of biodiversity and restoring degraded ecosystems. By changing our consumption habits and patterns, we can exert pressure so that environmental policies focus on reshaping social systems and basic production systems. (This includes social practices and cultural values, such as fostering regenerative ranching, which consists of recovering ecosystems' vital processes while offering the means for dignified living conditions in rural communities.) Taking the path toward conscious eating would make it possible to restore diverse habitats that have been damaged, and it would prevent continued land degradation while also presenting a potential solution for water scarcity issues.

Yes, we can all acknowledge that the necessary efforts to change course and create new trends are beyond one individual's capacity, but in our personal lives, we can move toward simplicity, which will allow us to be more generous with our surroundings. What we need to remember is that if this act of generosity toward the planet can be replicated among our family and social groups, then the "force of one" can become an incredibly powerful transformative agent.

AND IF I TURN A BLIND EYE?

Whenever I read this kind of information, I feel overwhelmed. On the one hand, the UN is saying the outlook doesn't look good for 2050. On the other, some experts deny these statements and offer scientific evidence to prove that everything is fine, and that soil degradation and air and water pollution are a natural process in the planet's evolution. There's also the other extreme of those who insist climate change is a ruse and that its only aim is to distract our attention as humans, as part of conspiracy theories and an alien invasion (as my relative regularly posts from the comfort of his hammock while enjoying his ocean view).

There are many environmental situations and problems that I don't understand very well or about which I'm not informed enough to reach my own conclusions. So, with a heavy heart, I wait for someone else to have enough courage and knowledge to do something about it. Hopefully, someone will invent a new kind of technology to change the trends of deterioration and degradation for the good of future generations… And then I return to my daily life with a pit in my stomach that has a numbing effect on me as I go about my regular activities. Surely, governments and organizations will do something, I think trustingly, and I focus once more on all those trivialities that usually take up my time. Sometimes, as part of my daily tasks, I come across activities and objects that harm the environment, but since I already feel a heavy weight on my shoulders, it's easier for me to bury my head in the sand and avoid my feelings of guilt. It's more comfortable to live in a state of denial, indifference, or resignation or to blindly trust that someone else will find a solution than it is to feel the pain from the part of the responsibility that corresponds to me. Many of us sleepwalk through life, apparently awake, but we do it automatically, without thinking, without feeling, losing more and more capacity to love and see ourselves reflected in the eyes of other people and creatures who coinhabit this planet with us. We go about our lives trying to forget that we are responsible for the world that was entrusted to us. It is ours to take care of—not to exploit. We start losing sight of the essence of what it is that makes us "human beings." So, with a knot in my throat that I don't know how to describe, I wonder: As a social group, how did we stray off a moral and spiritual path based on respect for the planet and all the beings that inhabit it?

It amazes me to see what some spiritual leaders such as Gandhi, the Dalai Lama, Saint Francis of Assisi, and others say—or have said—about caring for the environment. When I saw the movie "The Two Popes," I remembered that Pope Francis wrote an encyclical letter about the environment in 2015.[9] That same year, I received a bound version of that text as a Christmas gift from the environmental fund where I worked. Honestly, I hadn't read it, but after watching the movie, I was quite interested in hearing the Pope's opinion of the current situation. What first stood out to me is that the statements made in the *Laudato Si'* from 2015 are very similar to the conclusions the UN reached in 2019. For example, it says: *"We have not yet managed to adopt a circular model of production capable of preserving resources for present and future generations, while limiting as much as possible the use of non-renewable resources, moderating their consumption, maximizing their efficient use, reusing and recycling them..."* Perhaps if one of the UN researchers had read the encyclical in 2015, we would not have wasted four years talking about the need for a model of "environmental circularity."

One of Pope Francis's observations that made me reconsider the way I act when facing environmental challenges is the fact that, when I let things pass me by or turn a blind eye, it doesn't make me

---

[9] Encyclical letter *Laudato Si'* of the Holy Father Francis on care for our common home.

a better person. On the contrary, if I don't do anything about it, hoping that others find a solution, I'm numbing my soul. The encyclical points out that *"inasmuch as we all generate small ecological damage we are called to acknowledge our contribution, smaller or greater, to the disfigurement and destruction of creation."* So, as the saying goes, if we are not part of the solution, we are part of the problem, and, unfortunately, much of what we could do to contribute to solving the environmental crisis is thwarted by our lack of interest.

We have been conditioned by the industry and large corporations (which are only driven by their own financial benefit) to get short-term satisfaction without being morally or emotionally affected by the consequences these actions will have in the future or the suffering we cause others. *"A minority believes that it has the right to consume in a way which can never be universalized, since the planet could not even contain the waste products of such consumption."*[10] This is why we opt not to see those who live in miserable conditions and are most affected by our unrestrained and inequitable lifestyles. We must remember that the world population is estimated to reach 10 billion inhabitants by 2050 and that meeting the UN's proposed sustainable development goals is a humane and generous act that we are all equally responsible for. The goals are:

1) No poverty
2) Zero hunger
3) Good health and well-being
4) Quality education
5) Gender equality
6) Clean water and sanitation
7) Affordable and clean energy
8) Decent work and economic growth
9) Industry, innovation, and infrastructure

---

[10] Ibid.

10) Reduced inequalities

11) Sustainable cities and communities

12) Responsible consumption and production

13) Climate action

14) Life below water

15) Life on land

16) Peace, justice, and strong institutions

17) Partnerships for the goals

There is no more space—or time—for globalized indifference in the world. We should start to act like a society that is seeking the mutual benefit of its members, because we have a moral obligation to the world, to our fellow humans, and to the rest of the species who share the Earth with us.

It is also easier to turn a blind eye when animals, who don't have a voice, are treated cruelly to provide us with food and clothing or to test the adverse effects of our cosmetic products. As the Pope said, we are living in an age of consumerism that does not close the production cycle, as any balanced system would do, but rather that ends up filling the planet with the waste we throw out when it can't be reintegrated into the process. Not only do our productive processes create pollutants, but we also destroy stretches of forests, jungles, and aquifer layers to arrange the planet in accordance with our short-term needs and desires—once again—without thinking of the consequences this will have for ourselves, those in most need, and our children's children.

To turn these tendencies around, all we can do is speak the language of compassion, solidarity, and generosity with the world and all the beings that live here in this home that provides for us. If we don't, our time here on Earth will be seen as that of a vile thief of resources who was incapable of putting a limit on his immediate yearnings.

Fortunately, ecological awareness is growing among certain populations. A few weeks ago, I traveled back to my beloved Mexico, *lindo y querido*, and went to Coyoacán in southern Mexico City to eat some quesadillas. Before we sat down, we went over to a stand to buy mandarin juice, and I was very pleasantly surprised to see a sign that said they were not offering customers straws or lids for the cups in efforts to care for the environment. Where I live now, this wouldn't even happen by mistake. The first thing they do at many restaurants is bring you cups with straws. All in all, I know the Mexican conscience has been strongly interwoven with environmental care, and, in many places, it's common to see these types of actions. We have the responsibility but also the wonderful opportunity to value and take care of our planet's natural beauties. There are other countries, like Costa Rica, where this awareness is even greater, and people's respect for nature is even more deeply engrained. Most hotels and beaches in Costa Rica are built in harmony with their natural surroundings, and locals reflect their appreciation for the fruits of the Earth. However, on a global level, we have a lot to do, and small actions are the first step in making big changes.

Another piece of good news is that we don't have to keep waiting for someone to have a brilliant idea or propose an innovative technological solution. As consumers, we can do something about this by changing the way we behave as part of the production chain. These changes will save us and future generations from having to pay the high costs of environmental degradation.

Finally, we are the ones consuming the products that large companies sell. Think about it: These large companies spend millions of dollars on advertising campaigns and product engineering because their aim is to hook us and make us believe that life will be worthless if we don't buy what they're offering. Yes, these are the large companies that invest millions in developing the exact flavor and texture so we can't eat just one.

In the following chapters, I'll tell you about the constant bombardment of subliminal messages and the conditioning effects that we have repeated to the point of turning them into *truths*. The goal is to present information that helps you see a new horizon with fresh eyes or a light at the end of the tunnel, so you can stop sleepwalking and get back in touch with what makes us human. I'd like to invite you to read with an open mind and, if you have any questions, do the research you think is necessary and reach your conclusions.

It's important for this to be crystal clear: As consumers, we have the strength of millions. Without the cradle, the hand looking to rock it loses power.

TIP #2: What can you do?

✓ You can start by recognizing yourself as part of the problem, and then you can assume your responsibility.

✓ Analyze the impact that your decisions, behaviors, and consumption patterns have on the planet.

✓ Try to avoid products that include genetically modified ingredients because these agricultural practices threaten biodiversity. (I'll explain why later on.)

✓ In terms of food, imagine how a product reached your table. If another being suffered for it to get there, then analyze if it might be better to avoid it.

✓ Try to satisfy your hunger to around 80% and avoid eating until you feel full or like you are about "to burst."

✓ Consider that when you feel hungry it might actually be thirst or anxiety. Drink a glass of water and, to deal with the anxiety or worries, eat some crispy vegetables or fruit—such as carrots, jicama, cucumbers, or apples—or serve yourself a portion of unshelled pumpkin seeds.

‹~ 3 ~›

ARE YOU SURE?
THINK AGAIN

NUTRITION SCIENCE: PURE NUTRITIONISM?

S ome time ago, I had an initial session with a new client. This person told me she had intermittently followed the keto diet for many years as she fervently explained the malignance of carbohydrates. The keto (ketogenic) diet focuses on increasing the intake of foods that are rich in fat and protein and strictly reduces the intake of carbohydrates. She had read on the internet that certain fruits and vegetables are high in the latter macronutrient, and therefore, she voiced her need to completely restrict them from her eating plan. After listening to her for a few minutes, I asked her if she was clear about what carbohydrates were, and she answered that they were foods with a high content of "processed sugar and flour."

Yes, the world of eating has become a language of terms that we often never fully understand but that we repeat and repeat until creating a false reality in our minds that justifies the decisions about our lifestyles and, especially, about the way we eat. To make things even more confusing, nowadays, it's easy to hear comments in the gym like, "I read in a magazine that it's possible to lose weight by eating fewer carbs and more protein while being careful about how much saturated fat is in our food."

When I read Michael Pollan's book *In Defense of Food: An Eater's Manifesto*, I understood the relationship that we, as a modern society, have with food. One of the concepts this book puts forth is the term "nutritionism," which was coined by the Australian sociologist Gyorgy Scrinis. The term refers to the trend of understanding the relationship between 1) food and 2) our bodies, in terms of giving a nutritional value to the former to satisfy the chemical and nutritional needs of the latter. In short, it's reducing food to its nutrients, or pure reductionism. Nutritionism pushes us to understand what we eat as isolated nutrients, which makes our decisions about eating complicated. The suffix "-ism" is used to refer to an ideology based on doctrines, systems, schools, traditions, lifestyles, hierarchy, and scientific terms, among others, more so than on science itself (which only has authority through demonstration). For those of us who live our lives immersed in a certain ideology, it's hard to observe it and be aware of it. It's like trying to see the forest when we're standing in the middle of it. Pollan compares ideologies to the weather, saying how they're nearly impossible to get away from because of how pervasive they are.

Human beings organize life experiences into assumptions that we share as a society but that often have little or no foundation. Pollan says that, in the case of nutritionism, the widely shared assumption— which lacks scientific basis—is that the key to understanding a particular food is in its particular nutrients. Since nutrients are invisible, and therefore mysterious, the rest of us mere mortals leave it to the experts to explain "the hidden reality" of food.

So, according to the theory of nutritionism, we subject ourselves to the ideas that 1) the world we can see is not what's important and 2) to understand the invisible world, which our health depends on, we need help from experts who understand. To jumble things up even more, each expert has a favorite nutrient, and each nutrient has its moment of glory and of retribution. Like any ideology, nutritionism is based on dualistic thinking. There will always be a harmful nutrient that should be condemned and a vindicated nutrient that is sanctified…until the theories are updated and the experts redeem themselves with a "Sorry, we made a mistake" (which has been happening at a faster rate and, unfortunately, leaves us feeling lost in a sea of information that we don't understand). This promotes food trends, fads, and phobias that swing us on a pendulum that is oscillating faster and faster chasing after new discoveries and theories and, of course, the financial interests of a few. What should be clear to us is that the big beneficiary in the debate about nutrients is the food industry.

The history of our current relationship with food has its origins at the dawn of the 19th century when William Prout, an English doctor and chemist, identified the three macro components of food: proteins, fats, and carbohydrates, commonly known as macronutrients. In line with this discovery, in the mid 19th century, the German scientist Justus von Liebig spoke of the importance of minerals. He proposed the theory of metabolism—which explained life in terms of a handful of chemical nutrients—and declared that the mystery of nutrition had been solved. By the late 19th century and the early 20th century, it became evident that the set of chemicals proposed by Liebig was not enough to uphold his theories and explain diseases such as scurvy[11] or rickets.[12] Several years later, the Polish biochemist Casimir Funk identified some organic substances in fruits and vegetables, which he named by coining the term "vitamins" (composed of the Latin word for "life," *vita* and the chemical concept *amina*). Vitamins decked out nutrition science with more glamor and mystery, which helped confirm

---

[11] A disease caused by a vitamin C deficiency, which is characterized by a drop in blood quantity, bruise marks, gum ulcerations, and hemorrhages.

[12] A childhood disease caused by a lack of calcium, phosphorus, and vitamin D, which is characterized by bone deformation and muscle weakness.

that it belonged exclusively to the sphere of experts. This was how this new science, which only a few understood, opened a window of opportunity to a handful of groups that were interested in their own financial gain.

This struggle between nutrients has led modern society to such an extreme that, for example, edible products developed in factories claim to be healthier than foods grown from the Earth because their nutritional content has been designed by engineers and, according to the companies that aim to sell their products, they have the best combination of nutrients for human beings. Moreover, since the meat and dairy industries don't want to lose the boost from this consumer confusion, it's not out of the ordinary to find labels on industrialized products with some type of oxymoron,[13] like one of these, for example: "low-fat cheese," "hormone-free milk," or "*lean* red meat."

As human beings, we have been turned into the guinea pigs of modern times and the targets of advertising campaigns that benefit mega-corporations because, unfortunately, financial markets pressure corporations to the point that they feel obligated to maximize their profits in real time, without concern for the future or the generations to come. We are immersed in a frenzy around our eating caused by subliminal advertising, incomprehensible nutritional terms, official recommendations pushed by the financial interests of a few, and lies about the health benefits of processed edible products. And not only are we totally and undeniably confused, but the production and exploitation systems imposed on us by the industry make us sick and keep us depressed, overfed, and in search of the magical pill or easy solution that will bring us back to our ideal weight and health.

And what's going on is that we have lost sight of the simplest part of the equation: food. We have stopped eating authentic food

---

[13] A figure of speech that consists of combining two expressions with opposite meanings in the same structure. Etymologically, it is a word composed of two Greek terms whose meanings are "sharp" and "foolish." It's literal meaning is absurd and incoherent.

(which has minerals from the Earth and energy from the sun and, therefore, offers us life), and we have become focused on eating nutrients. And then things happen that are totally absurd. For instance, today, Americans' annual spending on diets and weight loss mechanisms is 50 times higher than the amount the UN allocates to programs to fight hunger. The tragedy is that—since nutritionism is backed by information we receive through mass media—as ordinary citizens, we believe it without questioning it and then turn it into a truth that's written in stone.

Once I heard Mark Bittman[14] say something that really stuck with me, and to bring this chapter to a close, I'd like to share this same idea with you: The mystery of nutritionism creates chaos, and this paves the way for the food industry and mega-corporations. They take their overly processed junk food and pump it with fiber and vitamins. Then, they tell us it's low in sodium, saturated fat, and cholesterol so they can sell it to us as a healthy product. And what's more, they get the backing of groups such as the American Heart Association (AHA) and the American Dietetic Association (ADA).

If we stop to think, doesn't it seem a little Dantean?

TIP #3: What can you do?

- ✓ Start appreciating food as a unit and not as isolated nutrients.
- ✓ We don't need to see or understand micronutrients. If we eat the food that has been with us throughout our evolutionary process as human beings, we can be sure that our nutritional requirements are covered.
- ✓ The foods that offer the greatest health benefits are those without packaging and, therefore, without labels highlighting their qualities.

---

14 U.S. journalist, author, and former columnist of *The New York Times*.

✓ Don't be misled by arguments and claims promoting a higher consumption of processed edible products. Remember, in these cases, the big beneficiary is the industry that promotes and sells them.

LAWS OR MECHANISMS OF MANIPULATION?

D
r. Marion Nestle tells a fascinating story in her book *Food Politics: How the Food Industry Influences Nutrition and Health.* In 1986, she was hired as an editorial advisor to develop the Surgeon General's nutrition policies, the "1988 Surgeon General's Report on Nutrition and Health." The aim of the publication was to show the relationship between diet and the chronic disease incidence. Dr. Nestle remembers how they made it very clear on her first day of work that she would need to follow certain rules, telling her that regardless of what she found in the studies she reviewed and compiled, under no circumstances could the policies suggest a reduction in the consumption of meat.

To understand this story, let's go back in time a little further. In the United States, in the late 1970s, the chronic disease incidence became the primary public health concern. The Senate Committee on Nutrition and Human Needs (which I'll just call "the committee" from now on) led by Senator George McGovern and originally formed to address malnutrition, decided to step in. By the 1950s, a group of epidemiologists and scientists had noticed that, during the war—when meat and dairy products were scarce and strictly rationed—the chronic disease incidence was very low, but when the armed conflict ended, the rate shot back up to pre-war levels. As a result of these observations, scientists concluded that the increase in fat and cholesterol (a waxy substance very similar to fat) from animal products was the cause of coronary diseases. This argument was called "the lipid hypothesis." By the 1970s, different specialists had also noticed that the coronary disease rate in societies with diets based heavily on animal products and processed foods was high, while in other cultures, with mainly plant-based diets, the rate was minimal. The committee took the conclusions from these studies, which seemed indisputable, and issued some guidelines to urge U.S. citizens to reduce the servings of red meat, eggs, and dairy products on their plates. This brilliant document was called: "Dietary Goals for the United States."

In a matter of weeks, a wave of criticism from the meat and dairy products industry fenced the committee in, and Senator McGovern (whose critical mass of voters was primarily made up of cattle ranch owners) was forced to step back. The committee's recommendations were promptly rewritten, and the suggestion to "reduce red meat and dairy products" literally changed to: "select foods from within the meat, fish, poultry and vegetable groups that are relatively low in fat, saturated fat, and cholesterol." Nutritionism made its triumphant entrance, sneaking the interests of a few in front of the good of society in general. Despite their obvious differences—in order to protect the industry—meat, poultry, and fish were grouped together as "a protein delivery system," and the cause of chronic disease was assigned a new villain: saturated fat. After this regretful disagreement between the government and the industry, Senator McGovern lost the next election, which sent a very clear message: "Leave the food industry alone."

Unfortunately, once the guidelines were published (previously approved by the industry, of course), the portions of animal products on consumers' plates remained unchanged, while other types of fat (like trans fats) were added alongside a long list of processed foods. The result? Coronary disease rates didn't go down, and overweight and obesity turned into an epidemic. Today, the coronary disease incidence is the same, but the number of deaths has, indeed, decreased—not as a result of dietary and lifestyle changes, but because of technological advancements in the field of medicine.

The use of nutritional terms to regulate U.S. dietary guidelines gave large corporations the chance to manipulate products and consumers' perceptions. The already empowered food industry took full control over dietary recommendations, and, today, it permits discussion only on nutrients—without mention of foods. And this was exactly the experience that Dr. Nestle had. The document she was put in charge of was intended to be published once every two years. Only the 1988 edition saw the light, however, since the terms and its scope were too complicated for daily life, and they created a false perception of the true nutritional value of foods. The space reserved for what we'd formerly simply known as "food" had been colonized by terms such as proteins, fats, carbohydrates, calories, vitamins, minerals, cholesterol, fiber, amino acids, and antioxidants, among others.

Another highly unfortunate event that illustrates the pressure the industry exerts on the entities and institutions whose function should be to secure society's health and well-being was when the National Academy of Sciences (NAS) analyzed the relationship between diet and cancer with the intention of issuing dietary recommendations. When this nonprofit organization published its results, it was very careful to suggest nutrients and not foods, as to avoid threatening anyone's financial interests. This is a clear example of how we live in an age in which nutrients have undoubtedly won the battle over food and, similar to what Pollan has explained, reductionism has the virtue of being both politically correct and intellectually thorough.

This might be the clearest example of the industry's power: Around the world, we have the false understanding that the U.S. Supreme Court is committed to making debate on public interests (both social and political) uninhibited, robust, open, and free of the fear of repercussions, even in controversial or potentially libelous cases. Yet, in dietary matters, there's a different reality. In the United States, no one can publicly suggest reducing the servings of a certain product because the affected associations and groups, which are protected by state laws, have the right to sue for defamation. To understand the intention of these laws, we need to go back to 1992, when the American Feed Industry Association (AFIA)—a lobbying group for the multi-million-dollar cattle feed and pet food industries—hired a law firm to draft model legislation against "discrediting foods," which would enable food manufacturers and producers to hold individuals responsible for criticizing their products. The bill was rejected on the federal level. However, due to pressure from the industry, 13 states (representing largely agricultural and ranching areas)[15] adopted this model legislation. These state laws are known as "veggie libel laws,"[16] and, in general, they allow the plaintiff (the industry) to impose punitive damage onto the defendant as well as attorney fees and any other financial harm that is brought about by their statements. It's common to find the following provisions in these state laws:

1. Individuals can be sued for presenting any type of information, including scientific hypotheses and opinions.

2. If someone discredits a product, anyone involved with the affected industry may come forward as a potential plaintiff.

And it was just a matter of time before someone fell into the trap… In April 1996, Oprah Winfrey organized a show called "Dangerous Foods" and invited the activist and animal rights defender Howard Lyman to speak about mad cow disease which, at the time, was a burning issue in the United Kingdom. On the program, Lyman insisted that the U.S. government had the obligation to ban the practice of feeding farm animals the remains of other animals. And the thing was, some theories about the origin of bovine spongiform encephalopathy (mad cow disease) indicated that it was caused by feeding cattle and other farm animals with animal remains and feces. Before this practice was outlawed, the remains of animals that died on

---

[15] Alabama, Arizona, Colorado, Florida, Georgia, Idaho, Louisiana, Mississippi, North Dakota, Ohio, Oklahoma, South Dakota, and Texas.
[16] They are also sometimes called "food libel laws" or "food-disparagement laws."

farms were used to make a variety of products, like candles and soaps, but what was left over—mainly the densest protein and the fecal matter—was ground into a brown powder that was used to supplement the animal feed. Oprah asked if there was any proof to back these statements up, and Lyman replied that it was a standard practice, which he had been part of several years ago when he managed a profitable agribusiness. Taken aback, Oprah reacted by exclaiming that this had stopped her in her tracks and she would never eat a hamburger again. This statement (whose effect is known as the "Oprah Crash" because it made the meat futures market plummet) sparked one of the dirtiest, most expensive, and longest legal battles in history when the Texas Beef Group sued Oprah and Lyman for a sum of $10.3 million under the Texas state law passed in 1995. When he found out about the lawsuit, Lyman said, "A funny thing can happen when you tell the truth in this country: you can end up getting sued."

Despite having won and getting the opportunity to state that freedom of expression had not only won the trial but also the battle, it's been speculated that the case cost Oprah and Lyman around one million dollars in legal fees. Not just anyone could pay this price, and so, once again, the industry made the rules of the game clear. The problem with these types of laws is that they restrict freedom of expression and also inhibit and limit individuals from showing their concerns about health risks, ethical implications, and the environmental impact of our current food system.

So, in a nutshell, what's going on is that our freedom of expression is limited by the pressure that a few exert to defend their financial interests. The industry manipulates the information we receive for their own benefit, and we are so immersed in nutritionism, so saturated that it becomes difficult to try to observe objectively and from outside of the hurricane's eye what, how, and why we eat what we eat.

Additionally, other factors that have covered our eyes are:

1. Recommendations from experts who are heavily influenced by the industry. According to Dr. Nestle, academia, research teams, and certain social groups receive significant funding from the food industry. In effect, sponsorship agreements are crucial since these resources are needed to carry on with research, but despite the existence of a vow of impartiality, the relationship between researchers and corporations calls the objectivity of these studies into question.

2. The constant bombardment of advertising that offers us a magical solution, a perfect nutrient, or the key to weight loss through multi-million-dollar advertising campaigns whose only aim is to convince us that we need the products the industry is selling.

3. Large corporations misuse science and information, and they have even won over the government with their political favors. The "revolving door" is quite common, which, as you'll remember, is the practice of politicians finishing their terms in office and then taking up important posts in lobbying groups (diverse interest groups that seek to influence decision-making) and vice versa. This puts the objectivity of how certain policies are administered into doubt.

Eating has become an act of faith, and we are standing in the middle of the crossfire in a battle between different edible products that fill our heads with false promises. If you still think it's important to ask where you'll get your protein from or if you're worried about eating some carbohydrates from your list of forbidden foods, then I'd like to invite you to keep reading so you can sort out this mess that we've been making by placing our salvation in the hands of experts on the invisible world of nutrients, by trusting that the actions of large corporations are laudable, and by believing that the government is here to protect us.

Myths and Legends

The illusion of truth

“ “**B**reakfast is the most important meal of the day.” This is something we've heard since we were kids, and our grandmothers, moms, and even our doctors have repeated it to us to the point of exhaustion. And they keep repeating it to us now that we are parents and concerned about our children's health. A few years ago, I went to a work breakfast where our charismatic host stressed to us guests several times that our mission was to read over the menu carefully and order the biggest dishes, alluding to this phrase that we have had tattooed on our chest from the day our first tooth started to show.

And so, we've obediently echoed it, generation after generation, among friends, from doctor to patient, or when recommending the key to leading a happy and healthy life to others. We repeat it with self-assurance, as if it were a decree inscribed in stone, but have you ever asked yourself why?

“Breakfast is the most important meal of the day” is one of the many phrases that has been etched onto our daily lives, but what's behind this absolute truth that's operating in the collective unconscious? The fascinating story behind this phrase is that it was coined by the U.S. doctor John Harvey Kellogg in the late 19th century due to his religious belief that having whole-grain flakes for breakfast would reverse the symptoms of different diseases—including indigestion. The cereal (actually created by James Caleb Jackson) and the brand known as Kellogg's were invented as part of a medical treatment based on the system of the recently formed Seventh-Day Adventists church.

Before this idea came about, breakfast didn't hold an important title, and, for most of the population, it consisted of oatmeal and leftovers from the meals they ate the day before. Throughout his medical career, Dr. Kellogg spoke of the harmful effects of digesting proteins and promoted a diet with higher amounts of carbohydrates. Since he was in favor of vegetarianism, his strategic objective was to oust animal protein. He focused on promoting a change in the breakfasts of well-to-do people, which consisted of eggs and meat. Together with his brother, Will Keith, he founded the Sanitas Foods Company in the late 19th century. Several years later, Will established his own company, which later became the Kellogg Company. The phrase was not only used for health and religious purposes, but in the early 20th century, the idea was also used to convince patients that the lighter and healthier their breakfasts were, the more efficient and productive their workdays would be. In the 1940s, boxed cereals started to be fortified with vitamins and, as a consequence of the period's advertising campaigns, a greater portion of the population started to give breakfast an important role.

A combination of the fear of indigestion plus religion, morals, and advertising propelled the phrase, but what consolidated the idea was the advertising campaign to sell bacon that was conceived and carried out by Mr. Edward Bernays, known as the father of public relations and advertising. Mr. Bernays asked the doctor from his agency to claim that a breakfast high in animal protein, consisting of bacon and eggs, was healthier than a light breakfast, and he sent this statement to 5,000 doctors to collect their signatures. Then, he got newspapers to publish the outcome of his petition as if it were presenting the results of a scientific study. This put bacon and eggs on the American table and gave greater weight to the idea that a large breakfast, rich in animal protein, was not only important but also a medical recommendation.

This was how the phrase that was coined by Dr. Kellogg to promote eating whole-grain flakes for breakfast, then massively promoted to sell Kellogg's cereals years later, and then further manipulated through marketing by Mr. Bernays to benefit his clients turned into one of the laws that no one dares to question today.

Often, we can find the true meaning of words in their etymological root. In English, "breakfast" means "to break the fast." The same is true in Spanish, *desayuno* means "to stop or leave (*des-*) the fast (*ayuno*)," and in French, *petit déjeuner* means "the small meal." Indeed, breakfast is an important meal because it's the way we end the fasting period that began after the last meal of the previous day. This fast is a time for our bodies to carry out detoxification, recovery, and restoration processes. Traditionally speaking, after a fasting period, the first ingestion should be moderate in order to be gentle on the body's systems and organs that carried out their renovation processes. Yet, today, not only do we ignore its etymological meaning, but, through constant and conditioned repetition, we have turned the first meal of the day into a small feast, eating as if there were no tomorrow. Consequently, if we think of the true meaning of breakfast, not only are we believing this slogan as an unquestionable truth—a slogan that Dr. Kellogg invented, that his brother exploited to sell his products, and that an advertising genius used for the financial gain of a few— but we are also eating it in portions that were never part of the original intention. This is just one example that shows how many of the truths we take for granted are actually just sayings and opinions that we have repeated enough times to make them into law.

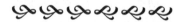

The false truth we know best: "We need animal protein as part of every meal."

As parents, we're always trying to make sure our children get the proper amount of protein so that they'll grow up strong and healthy. If we don't do this, our neighbors, friends, and relatives will start to raise their eyebrows and shake their fingers at us. Yet, where does this strongly ingrained conviction come from?

In the mid 19th century, basing his statements on studies by Dr. Prout, Mr. Liebig (the German scientist whom I mentioned in the previous chapter) declared protein a "master nutrient" because he considered it to be the key factor for growth in animals. By the late 19th century, many countries were facing a health crisis caused by two factors: malnutrition (especially in social classes with scarce resources) and the infectious disease rate, which primarily afflicted the malnourished population. At the time, governments had the job of promoting the consumption of a higher number and greater variety of foods. These perfect circumstances between 1) new discoveries in nutrition and 2) the population's state of health laid the foundations for building our current food system around Liebig's favorite nutrient. At this time, many societies had been devastated by financial crises and wars, and they were hit hard by the scarcity of fruits and vegetables. In extreme situations, foods with a high protein content have, indeed, made the difference between life and death for thousands of children and adolescents, which is why the government tasked itself with making them financially accessible for the entire population. This door opened an ideal opportunity for the food industry: produce, sell more products, and yield higher profits. Having the government's moral and financial support along with the suggestion to include a wide variety of foods in the diet, the industry wasted no time in producing and providing the highest amount of food possible. It also took advantage to design and produce edible products—all with a high content of added salt, sugar, and fat.

From the early 20ᵗʰ century until the end of World War II, the rates of malnutrition and infectious diseases went down, but the way was paved for illnesses related to diet and lifestyle: chronic diseases (obesity, cardiovascular diseases, cancer, and diabetes, among others). By the end of the 1960s, scientific studies had made it clear that these illnesses were the result of abusing foods with a high content of saturated fats (mainly from animal products), salt, and sugar, and it was time to change the message from eating more to eating less. With the common well-being in mind, the U.S. government made an effort to relay this knowledge to society (remember the story about Senator McGovern). The food industry already had the necessary means to manipulate the government, however, and—of course—it wouldn't spare any efforts or resources to keep gaining ground. There were so many interests at play that the government had no choice but to yield to this coercion and, to avoid affecting the industry's financial interests, nutritional guidelines incorporated terms about nutrients that were unintelligible for ordinary citizens, thus making food regulations the clearest example of pure nutritionism. Additional pressure led to eliminating certain words such as "limit" and substituting them with others that weren't quite as harsh, such as "moderate." As consumers, we were left adrift, making us easy prey for the huge wave of misinformation and deceptive advertising practices. To date, the truth is veiled by pressure from the industry, and as consumers we are at the mercy of nutritional trends, fads, and phobias, watching as one particular micronutrient comes about one day and, the next day, another.

Due to excessive food production, many countries around the world have a surplus supply—simply put, we are drowning in food. For example, food production in the U.S. (not considering what is earmarked for export) is enough to offer every person double the amount of their daily calorie requirements. Also, today it has been identified with great clarity that malnutrition can go both ways: over-nourishment is just as problematic as under-nourishment. It is quite easy to detect which countries have a food supply that is greater than the demand and, therefore, face the serious problem of over-nourishment: all you have to do is analyze overweight and obesity rates. And, when it comes to the issue of excess, everything indicates that much of the world is following in the footsteps of the Standard American Diet (SAD).

While the promotion and sponsorship of animal protein was an excellent mechanism for putting an end to malnutrition in a period of hunger, crisis, war, and infectious diseases, the excessive amounts that we eat today are counterproductive to our health. (Of course, this is referring to societies that have a surplus supply of food.) Moreover, according to Dr. Bruce Ames from the Children's Hospital Oakland Research Institute (CHORI), foods that treat short-term survival situations (those that are high in calories, such as animal proteins) in most cases do not offer us long-term health because they are deficient in micronutrients such as vitamins, minerals, and antioxidants, to mention a few. The greatest concerns in public health are chronic diseases resulting from lifestyle choices and diets with a very high caloric content and, sadly, our children are suffering the consequences. What kind of quality of life can the kids who already have these types of diseases expect to have? And even worse, what country is going to have the millions of dollars in resources to cover health expenses when today's children are adults?

And let's not forget, this is not only happening in the U.S. For example, my home country of Mexico has the highest rates of child obesity—a statistic that should shake us to the core. Don't you think we should take urgent measures as parents? It is unacceptable to keep living as if there's nothing that we can do or hoping that the situation will go away like magic. And the problem is that the industry has orchestrated infinite advertising gimmicks and engineered our food in order to hold us captive as customers, meaning no one is spared… The industry invests billions of dollars a year in research, lobbying, marketing, and misleading advertising to make us believe that their products will solve our problems, and, unfortunately, the need to include a portion of animal protein in each meal is included in this series of deceptions. Moreover, a big problem with including so much animal protein in our daily servings is that we don't put foods such as fruit, vegetables, and legumes on our plates or our children's plates, even though these are what provide us with the ideal chemical compounds for our long-term health.

If food guidelines and recommendations were honest and not compromised by the industry, they would clearly specify that in this age of surplus supplies of food, human beings should 1) eat less, 2) include more fruit, vegetables, legumes, whole grains, seeds, and nuts in every meal, and 3) limit their portions of meat, eggs, and dairy products to minimal quantities.

Just like that, without mincing words….

The master deception

Remember the marketing campaign "got milk?" that featured famous actors, models, and athletes photographed with a milk mustache? This campaign, which is incredibly aggressive and costly, started in the nineties with the goal of reverting the declining sales and commercialization of dairy products. The money to pay for it comes from the "check-off deduction" that I mentioned a few chapters ago. The impact that these kinds of campaigns have on consumers' perception gives mass media the power to create collective truths like the one supporting that "cow milk is the best source of calcium for human beings,"[17] which associations like the U.S. National Dairy Council (NDC) promotes. Once again, this paves the way for nutritionism as the source of a wave of misinformation surrounding yet another micronutrient that has come to our rescue: calcium.

It's true that the editors of print and digital media are just as misinformed as their readers when it comes to nutrition-related matters stemming from the industry's manipulation. (Media outlets such as *The New York Times, Business Week, Men's Health, Pediatrics, WebMD*, and *The Wall Street Journal*, among others, have published thousands of contradictory articles on the topic.) We've been misinformed that including enough calcium in our diets will make our bones strong and healthy. Actually, it's much more likely that the problem with this nutrient is not how much we ingest but rather how much we lose and the reasons why this happens in our bodies.

In his book *The China Study: Startling Implications for Diet, Weight Loss, and Long-Term Health*, Dr. T. Colin Campbell presents more than 8,000 statistical correlations between diets and diseases, which is why it is considered one of the best reference points for studying the consequences of including animal protein in our diets. Even though this study's results are statistically significant (the probability of getting the same results if the studies are repeated is high and the probability that the correlations are random is low), it's worth clarifying that correlation does not imply causation. That is, there is no scientific basis for determining that one variable is the cause of the other. Yet, this doesn't mean the correlations are not useful: well-interpreted, they can be a starting point for studying the origin of the relationships between the observed variables. The high number of correlations in this project offers relational patterns of variables as complex as diet, health, lifestyle, the risk of contracting certain diseases—such as

---

[17] https://www.nationaldairycouncil.org/content/2015/science-summary-dairy-and-peak-bone-mass

osteoporosis—that can be used to channel scientific studies and analyses. In short, the correlations show that something is, indeed, going on, but they do not offer the scientific explanation of the causes. Let me be clear that if you are interested in understanding the basis of the observed relationships, then the correlation of variables I share below won't be quite enough. In this case, I'd like you to know that all I'm intending to do is present information that I've been able to review and that has seemed relevant to me.

In his book, Dr. Campbell explains that there tends to be more osteoporosis in countries that have a higher intake of dairy products. The U.S., New Zealand, Sweden, the United Kingdom, Holland, Finland, Canada, Australia, and countries from northeast Europe are the primary consumers of calcium in the form of dairy products, and they are also the countries that have higher rates of bone fractures and osteoporosis. Meanwhile, South Africa (and other African countries), Papua New Guinea, Singapore, and China (although the trend is changing toward China being the number one consumer in years to come) have the lowest rates of dairy consumption, and they are cataloged among the countries with fewer cases of bone fractures and osteoporosis. Likewise, in 1992, Yale University School of Medicine carried out a review analyzing the relationship between protein ingestion and hip fracture rates. The data were taken from 34 independent studies conducted in 16 countries, and the results were published in 29 peer-reviewed research reports. This meta-analysis established a correlation of 70% between the rate of hip fractures and the presence of animal protein in the nutritional practices. Along the same lines, a few years ago, the journal *Pediatrics* published a review of a meta-analysis of 58 studies in which no relationship could be found between the consumption of dairy products and bone health. This paper determined that exercise is more important for strengthening bones than an increase in calcium intake.[18]

Just as there is not a scientific explanation to uphold that consuming lactose can cause osteoporosis (despite the statistical studies that show a correlation), in her book *Food Politics,* Dr. Nestle also makes it clear that there is no scientific basis proving that consuming dairy helps fight it either (or at the very least, reduce it). Despite this lack of scientific evidence, the U.S. Department of Agriculture (USDA) supports the claim that dairy products—in particular—improve bone health.[19] The USDA is the division of the U.S. federal government that, firstly, is in charge of developing and implementing livestock and agricultural policies and, secondly, oversees the development of nutrition guidelines for the country's population. Its main goal is to secure the benefit and financial growth of the agroindustry (including products such as corn and sugar), which is why its responsibility of developing food policies has been highlighted as a clear case of conflict of interest.

If you've heard that dairy products help improve bone health, ask the person who told you this where you can find the information backing this statement up—not recommendations but rather the scientific support. Remember, "suggestions" from government agencies or research institutes are not enough. What we're looking for is the scientific basis, and, if it exists, we'll want to know who funded the study.

Moreover, in contrast with vegetable proteins, animal proteins have a higher concentration of the amino acids cysteine and methionine. (We'll talk about vegetable proteins and amino acids in a few chapters.) When they are digested and metabolized, these amino

[18] Lanou, Amy Joy, et al., "Calcium, Dairy Products and Bone Health in Children and Young Adults: A Reevaluation of the Evidence," 115 *Pediatrics* (2005):736-43; ABC News Online, "Conventional Wisdom on Milk Questioned," March 7, 2005.
[19] https://www.choosemyplate.gov/eathealthy/dairy/dairy-nutrients-health

acids produce a sulfur radical as the precursor of sulfuric acid (acid-forming sulphate ion) that should be removed by the kidneys. It has been demonstrated that there is a correlation of 84% between the consumption of animal products and acid excretion through the urinary tracts. A great many studies (the first dates back to 1880 and was documented in 1920) conclude that animal protein increases acid in the blood and tissue. Accordingly, the body uses calcium from the bones to neutralize this acidity. Since 1970, research has demonstrated and detailed the causes of a calcium increase in urine due to consuming animal protein. Some medical studies have discovered that, upon duplicating the ingestion of animal protein, calcium in urine increases by 50%.[20] In short, the body taking calcium from the bones as a mechanism for neutralizing the acidity generated by foods of animal origin has been considered a plausible explanation.

Despite not having scientific support to prove the causes, wouldn't it seem that something doesn't make sense about the assertion that "dairy products = healthy bones"?

Drinking milk from another species in the quantities we drink in this day and age—an idea that, unfortunately, has been reinforced by our doctors and nutritionists—is a very recent phenomenon in human history. Several years ago, an evolutionary biologist from Colorado State University, Dr. Loren Cordain, pointed out that if milk were indeed an important factor for bone health, then the bone structure of our ancestors, who did not have access to this food, should have been fragile. Yet, Dr. Cordain found that the bones of distant generations were robust and resistant to fractures. Similarly, other analyses performed on the skeletons of post-menopausal women from the 18th and 19th centuries demonstrated that they had stronger and healthier bones than modern women in the same age range.

---

[20] Studies funded by the Atkins Center.

Everything seems to indicate that the amount of calcium we consume is one of the least significant elements on the list of essential requirements for keeping our bones healthy, and there is not enough evidence to conclude that cow milk helps human beings build stronger bones. Moreover, our bodies can absorb only a percentage of the calcium from milk, and this absorption rate depends on the presence of other minerals such as magnesium. According to recent studies, the calcium absorption from cow milk is an estimated 32%.

What no one can deny is that the dairy product industry, like the rest of the food industry, has invested millions of dollars in subliminal advertising, in efforts to influence the government, and in making arrangements with nutrition experts to declare that cow milk is "nature's perfect food." And if you think the dairy industry's power and influence don't extend beyond U.S. borders, think again. In Latin America, for example, governments (like Mexico's) continue to suggest dairy products as an important part of our diets even though Latinos have one of the highest rates of lactose intolerance,[21] affecting 50% of the population.

---

[21] Woteki, C.E., et al., "Lactose malabsorption in Mexican-American adults," *American Journal of Clinical Nutrition* 30 (1977): 470–75.

HAPPY FARMS AND GOLDEN FIELDS

I am not part of an animal defense group, and I'm far from considering myself an activist on the issue. I'm an average human, mom, wife, and careerwoman, with lots of dreams and a great desire to change the course of the planet, just like thousands of women around the world. But I do feel the weight of my part of the responsibility in terms of environmental deterioration, and I also hurt for the thousands of animals that are killed in order to reach our tables.

I haven't had the opportunity to spend time with a cow, a pig, or a chicken, but I've seen videos on Facebook of cows having fun with a ball, pigs playing hide-and-seek, and chickens running up to a boy for a hug. It has also been demonstrated that, when separated from their calves, cows feel a deep sense of melancholy that is very similar to the depression we feel as human beings; that pigs are so intelligent that, along with dolphins, they are capable of understanding how mirrors work; and that chickens can reason through deduction, a characteristic of species with a certain level of self-awareness.

ॐ॰ॐ॰ॐ॰ॐ॰ॐ॰ॐ

What are Concentrated Animal Feeding Operations?

Concentrated Animal Feeding Operations (CAFOs) are spaces where around 1,000 "animal units"[22] are concentrated for over 45 days

---

[22] Nearly all the definitions refer to a cow weighing around 100 pounds, including unweaned calves. Each animal unit is fed with approximately 25 pounds of dry fodder a day. One thousand animal units is equal to 1,000 cows; 700 cows used by the dairy industry; 2,500 pigs weighing over 55 pounds; 125,000 chickens; or 82,000 laying hens.

a year. In the U.S. alone, 450,000 industrial farms have been registered. CAFOs dominate the world's animal production industry because they provide a low-cost source of animal products. This makes it nearly impossible for family farms, local farms, and farms with regenerative livestock practices to compete in the market.

CAFOs have an impact that, unfortunately, is hidden from us as consumers. And they've been hiding it from us as a marketing stunt to 1) keep us from feeling bad about the standard practices at these sites and 2) continue to increase our consumption of animal products. And, as in any equation, the higher the consumption of animal products, the higher the number of CAFOs worldwide. These confinement sites defend themselves in the name of "efficiency," but their claims are false. The reality is that producing animal proteins with the objective of covering 100% of the world population's nutritional needs is highly inefficient, especially in a world where over 1 billion people go hungry. It would seem that animal products produced at these sites are cheap, but CAFOs end up costing us a lot of money: 1) in subsidies for the industry (paid with our taxes), 2) in higher medical bills, since they represent a health risk (which I'll describe below), 3) because land loses value in areas close to these sites (due to the long-term environmental damage they cause), and 4) because we, along with our children and their children, are also the ones who will pay the environmental costs of cleaning the water, soil, and air.

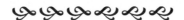

Bioaccumulation

Throughout our history, human beings have created and/or manipulated more than 80,000 chemical compounds that we are now exposed to. Despite the numerous benefits that chemical products have contributed to humanity, their polluting effects in this era—which has the highest chemical use in all of human history—represent a serious problem all over the world. Recent studies have detected more than 200 toxic chemicals in umbilical cord blood (fire retardants, plastics, additives, and pesticides have been found). The mother's womb should be a sterile environment, free of any of these compounds. We've been overtaken by our exposure to them, however, and the reality is that, from the day they're born, our children are already carrying a significant toxic load in their bodies. Many of these chemical compounds—like DDT[23], which was developed as a modern synthetic insecticide in the 1940s and, due to mounting evidence of its environmental and toxicological effects, was banned in the U.S. in 1972— are very persistent in the environment; they remain in the soil and can travel long distances in the upper atmosphere. They accumulate in the fatty tissues of the animals we eat, and also in our bodies. We bioaccumulate them, we pass them on to our children, and they continue to accompany us from one generation to the next.

The term *bioaccumulation* is made up of the prefix "bio-" (relating to life) and the word "accumulation" (the gathering or adding of one thing to another that contributes to the same effect). Together, they mean "the accumulation of harmful chemical compounds like pesticides, DDT, PCBs[24], dioxins[25], and mercury in a living organism." An organism bioaccumulates when it absorbs substances quicker than it can use them or eliminate them—that is, when more are coming in than are going out. The longer the organism takes to eliminate the

---

[23] Dichloro-diphenyl-trichloroethane (DDT) is classified as a probable human carcinogen by U.S. and international authorities.

[24] Polychlorinated biphenyls (PCBs) are persistent organic pollutants that—even with discontinued use—still pollute the environment and cause serious problems for human health.

[25] Dioxins are unwanted by-products of a wide range of processes including the manufacturing of some herbicides and pesticides. They are persistent environmental pollutants with highly toxic potential that accumulate in the fatty tissue of animals (mainly dairy products, fish, and shellfish).

substances (higher bioaccumulation), the higher the risk of chronic poisoning, even when the levels of the substance in the environment are not very high. The term was originally used in reference to aquatic organisms: A small fish absorbs a certain quantity of toxic substances directly from the environment. When a larger fish eats this small fish, the big fish bioaccumulates the chemical compounds contained in the fish it ate. If an even larger fish repeats this process, then its organism will bioaccumulate the toxic substances and compounds from the fish it ate, which, at the same time, had already received an additional load of pollutants from the smallest fish. The higher the trophic level[26] in the food chain, the higher concentration of harmful chemical compounds. The reason you hear the recommendation to eat only small fish nowadays (to avoid consuming tuna, for example) is because bioaccumulation in large fish has become an issue of concern for medical and scientific communities.

Some of the industrial and chemical residues that are routinely found in industrialized products of animal origin are antibiotics, pesticides, chemicals, and trace elements (minor bio-elements that are present in minute quantities in living beings that—in both their absence and excess—can be harmful to the organism). These residues produce an accumulative effect in human beings and other species. As human beings we already absorb toxic substances found in the environment and the objects we come into contact with (insecticides, medicines, cleaning products, clothing, cosmetics, furniture, carpets, swimming pools, air conditioners, etc.), but when we ingest animal products that have accumulated chemicals, toxic substances, and heavy metals, the load of compounds that are harmful to our bodies becomes exponential.

---

[26] The position of an organism in the food chain.

Below, I briefly describe two pollutant substances that we find in animal products (antibiotics and pesticides) that have a bioaccumulation effect on human beings.

Antibiotics

Since it deals with confined areas with high concentrations of animals, manure, urine, and carcasses and aims to avoid financial loss, the livestock industry takes measures to prevent any possibility of infection that could cause the premature death of these animals. For this same reason, at industrial farms, a huge number of antibiotics are prophylactically administered. (It's estimated that around 80% of the total production of antibiotics is used at these sites.) The purpose of giving these animals antibiotics as a preventative measure is to promote their quick growth and keep them alive long enough to reach the weight and size that will give them their maximum value. That's to say, it is also a strategy for maximizing profits in less time. There's still debate, but some scientific communities believe this practice, together with the indiscriminate use of antibiotics in human medicine, is one of the primary causes of microbial resistance (resistance to antibiotics) worldwide. A great many studies conclude that the practice of administering antibiotics to animals produced for human consumption can result in the development of this resistance and also in the disturbance of intestinal flora—consequently making it a risk for people's health. Here's a question to reflect on: If you knew exactly how many antibiotics were administered to the cow, would you feed a piece of its meat to your children or give them a glass of its milk to drink?

Pesticides

In order to talk about the damage caused by pesticides, first I have to talk about hormones. Hormones are molecules that act as the body's chemical messengers: they control and activate numerous functions and processes (like appetite, growth and development, blood pressure, energy use and storage, and reproduction). Hormones are very powerful compounds that travel through the bloodstream to the organs and tissues, and they cause vital changes on a cellular level. The endocrine system glands (adrenal, thyroid, thymus, and pancreas, to mention a few) are in charge of producing and secreting hormones. Some examples of hormones are insulin, cortisol, the growth hormone, testosterone, and estrogens. When these hormones are not properly balanced, this is called an endocrine system disorder.

Pesticides and certain chemical compounds have effects on the human body because of their properties that imitate endogenous hormones (those the human body produces naturally), which makes them one of the main causes of the endocrine system's disruption. Because they have structures similar to hormones, pesticides can access cells' DNA[27] and "super-activate" certain functions and processes in the body. Likewise, while the hormones our bodies produce are used and later naturally discarded, these "artificial hormones" interfere with the enzymes that facilitate their excretion. This causes hormone levels to shoot up and stay elevated for long periods.

Some conclusions from experiments on lab animals have demonstrated that pesticides:

1. Perform estrogenic activities. Estrogens play a key role in developing female physical characteristics and reproductive functions, including breast and uterus growth and menstrual cycle regulation. Men also produce estrogens, but in much lower quantities. However, high estrogen levels are a problem for both men and women because they can cause cardiovascular diseases; premature aging; obesity; hyperthyroidism; testicular tumors; problems with insulin

---

[27] DNA stands for "deoxyribonucleic acid," which is the chemical name of the molecule that contains the genetic instructions for the development and functioning of living beings.

production; and digestive, kidney, and liver problems. They can even set off some autoimmune diseases.

2. Create imbalances in the hormone levels produced by the thyroid gland that, in the early stages of pregnancy, can compromise the baby's neurological development.

3. Play an important role in learning disorders as well as in children's development and behavior as a result of their neurotoxic effects.

ᢒᢇ ᢒᢇ ᢒᢇ ᢇᢓ ᢇᢓ ᢇᢓ

Environmental degradation

Another consequence of having large concentrations of animals, manure, urine, and carcasses is the tremendous damage they cause to the planet's ecosystems and natural resources:

Water

Just think…these sites produce millions of tons of manure each year. How would you manage those millions of tons of manure? One of the easiest ways to get rid of this waste is to throw it in the water. Accordingly, the U.S. Environmental Protection Agency (EPA) has issued certain environmental regulations, such as the obligation to develop plans for managing residual waters. The plan these farms use most involves anaerobic lagoons or manure lagoons. Yet, it turns out that these approaches have not only been inefficient, but they have also strongly contributed to environmental and health problems globally. Without enough oxygenation, these lagoons produce methane and nitrous oxide. Due to its number of CAFOs, the United States has the highest methane emissions of any country in the world. As a result of the mismanagement of these excrements, it's common for areas with a higher concentration of CAFOs to experience an average of 20 to 30 serious water quality problems that affect both human beings and wildlife as well as diverse water systems such as groundwater flows, streams, rivers, lakes, and oceans.

The two main contributors to the water pollution caused by these farms are 1) soluble nitrogen compounds, which accumulate for decades in groundwater and cause human diseases, and 2) phosphorous, which causes the exponential growth of algae and, therefore, an oxygen deficit in aquifers, creating extensive dead zones in bodies of water. However, these farms also produce additional pollutants such as solid material (fur, feathers, and carcasses); pathogens (microorganisms that are capable of causing diseases); salts; trace elements (mainly arsenic); compounds such as carbon dioxide, methane, sulfuric acid, nitrous oxide and ammonia, and—as we've seen—antibiotics, hormones, and pesticides. These CAFO practices produce such large quantities of pollutants that they seriously threaten sources of drinking water all over the world.

Air

CAFOs also contribute to air pollution, since they release different types of particles and gas into the atmosphere, such as ammonia, hydrogen sulfide, nitrous oxide, and methane. As you might imagine, the main cause of these gas emissions is the decomposing manure that is stored in large quantities. Poultry farms release large quantities of ammonia from fermenting hen droppings, while all animal feces let off hydrogen sulfide that, beyond having a strong odor, is also potentially harmful to human health and the planet's health. Some CAFOs dispose of manure through other unhygienic and potentially infectious practices like spraying fields. (They basically put the manure in a machine that sprays it onto open fields. You tell me…)

Climate Change

Agriculture—including industrial farms, forestry, and other land uses are cataloged globally as the second-largest contributor of greenhouse gases that alter the atmosphere. They are known as greenhouse effect gases (carbon dioxide [CO_2], methane [CH_4], nitrous oxide [N_2O], and fluorinated gases) because they accumulate in the Earth's atmosphere where they absorb and emit infrared radiation. This causes an increase and retention of heat in the atmosphere.

Carbon dioxide (CO_2), which is derived from the burning of fossil fuels such as coal and petroleum and—to a lesser extent—from deforestation for agricultural purposes, is the primary cause of climate change. Methane gas (CH_4) is the second leading cause, and, specifically, confined livestock contributes 30% of the emissions of anthropogenic origin of this particular greenhouse effect gas (of which 17% is produced from manure management and the remaining 83% is caused by gases that are produced during ruminant digestion—intestinal fermentation). If no changes are made, methane emissions are expected to increase 60% by 2030. Known as laughing gas, nitrous oxide (N_2O) is about 300 times more potent than carbon dioxide when it comes to trapping heat in the atmosphere, where it remains for over 100 years before disintegrating. The largest producer of nitrous oxide is agriculture, particularly fertilized soil and animal manure. Although it comprises roughly 6% of greenhouse gas emissions, it has risen 30% in the last four decades. Experts say that the impact of laughing gas on the climate is no joke.

If we continue to alter the atmospheric composition, then the environmental, social, health, and financial repercussions could be catastrophic on a global level. (High concentrations of persistent, bioaccumulative toxic chemical substances have been predicted.) Moreover, the intensive agriculture that is necessary to feed this number of confined animals depends on a high use of fossil fuels: from nitrogen-based fertilizer synthesis to petroleum-based chemical products (pesticides and herbicides). The use of nitrogen-based fertilizers for soil treatment produces three-quarters of the nitrous oxide emissions, which also contributes to the rise in greenhouse gas effects.

The soil erosion and deterioration caused by CAFOs and the intensive agriculture that is necessary to feed this number of animals are also factors that significantly contribute to climate change. Industrial farms decrease the fertility of soil and alter its composition, causing carbon dioxide to be released into the atmosphere.

The only way to reverse the dangerous effects of climate change—which, as we saw, result from altering the composition of atmospheric gases—is 1) to reduce greenhouse gas emissions and 2) to restore soils, forests, and marine ecosystems to facilitate the capturing or "sequestration" of carbon from the atmosphere. Some experts claim we could rapidly and successfully reverse the effects of climate change by reducing the causes of these emissions and simultaneously regenerating our soils and terrestrial and marine ecosystems.

❧ ❧ ❧ ❧ ❧ ❧

The cruelty of industrial farms

There is still no legislation to regulate how animals at these confinement sites should be treated, and, consequently, what takes place inside their walls is truly cruel and inhumane.

In the U.S. alone, around 9 billion animals are killed for human consumption each year. If we were to line up all these animals, they would go from the Earth to the Moon five times. According to statistics from the World Economic Forum and Faunalytics, the global figure reaches 53 billion animals. If the number of animals we kill each year doesn't shock you, maybe the treatment they receive will. Below,

I present descriptions from a video that addresses the abuse they are subjected to during their time on industrial farms. This video has a significant amount of violent content, but if you want to see it with your own eyes, the link is in the footnote.[28]

Here, I'll simply summarize what is discussed so you can learn about some of the practices that are common due to a lack of regulation. I should warn you that the content is hard to take in, and if you don't feel ready to read it right now, go ahead and skip the next five paragraphs:

Pigs are truly smart and affectionate animals, and so it's awful that, on industrial farms, they live in cages that are so cramped that they can barely move. Some present symptoms of insanity due to the stress, abuse, and lack of mental stimulation. When they're born, piglets are castrated and their tails are mutilated—without anesthesia—and if they get sick or don't grow enough, they're killed by being slammed against the ground or put in gas chambers. The piglets that survive are locked up in confined spaces where they will never see the light of day or the freshness of grass. Their short lives will end when they turn six months old, which is the age at which they're sent to the slaughter plant to be hung by their back legs, receive very painful electrical shocks, and have their throats slit so they will die by bleeding to death.

Chicken are animals with unique personalities, like dogs and cats, but unfortunately some practices that would be prohibited with dogs and cats are allowed with these animals. When chicks are born on poultry farms, the males are separated from the females. Since males won't lay eggs, they are killed on the first day of their lives by being placed on conveyor belts that lead to a grinding machine. In the case of the females, their beaks are partially sliced off (which, by the way, are incredibly sensitive), and then they are packed into cages that are so small that they can barely move and can never fully spread

---

[28] https://www.youtube.com/watch?time_continue=571&v=pNxcylWLEH8&feature=emb_logo&has_verified=1

their wings. The constant rubbing against the metal bars makes their wings lose their feathers and cripples their feet.

Chickens and turkeys that are raised for meat have been genetically selected to grow so large that it's common for their legs, whose bones are extremely fragile, to break because they can't support their own weight. When this happens, due to a lack of individual veterinary care, the birds will lie on the feces-packed floors with broken legs, unable to move until the moment they die. If they are lucky, a farm worker will break their necks to save them from a slow and painful death. Many of these birds have heart problems and live with chronic pain. When they're sent to the slaughter plant, their heads are inserted into metal cones and their throats are also slit so they bleed to death, fighting for their lives.

Cows are such intelligent animals that they can remember a person's face for years. When they are free and have a reason to be happy, they'll jump in the air when they're excited. Cows usually have a "best friend" and are very selective when choosing a group of cows to spend time with. On dairy farms, cows are mutilated, without anesthesia; they get their horns and tails cut off and are also branded with a hot iron. These cows spend their entire lives standing on filthy floors or crammed into mud lots. In some cases, because of the hormones they're administered along with the suction effect of the milking machines, their udders grow so much that they drag on the floor (yes, that same disgusting, nauseating floor). Several times a day and without any cleaning process, their dirty udders are connected to the milking machines. (That's right, imagine what you might find in the milk.) On these dairy farms, cows are artificially inseminated on an ongoing basis, and when the calves are born, they are cruelly separated from their mothers, which causes a deep sense of sadness in both of them. (It has already been proven that all mammals have affective bonds that are generated in the limbic brain.) Once separated, male calves are killed, and the females are prepared to set off on the same path as their mothers.

Fish have different personality types and are very social beings. Their skin is extremely sensitive to water movement, so they also feel pain like any other animal, only they don't have vocal cords that allow them to emit sounds. Fish endure tremendous cruelty. Many are cut into pieces when still conscious and others are confined into spaces that are so small that it becomes hard for them to breathe—in part because of the number of fish that share the space, but also because of the amount of excrement that makes it impossible to move. There is highly significant collateral damage from overfishing that affects all marine ecosystems: many endangered species are direct victims of these types of unsustainable practices.

Naturally, producers don't want consumers to find out what's really going on at these sites, and they fill our screens and print media with images of happy cows, pigs, and farmers. Nothing could be further from the truth. In addition to being big polluters, industrial farms are places that cause a great deal of pain and suffering…pain and suffering that we later bring to our tables to offer to the people we love the most. Again, I can't help but wonder: How numb must our souls be to allow other sentient beings to be treated so cruelly and to suffer their entire lives so they can reach our tables as the main dish?

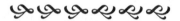

What do these animals eat?

Of the cereals, legumes and grains that are produced in the U.S. (mainly corn, soybeans, barley, and wheat), 77% are used as raw material for feed pellets, the primary food for industrialized animals. These crops, especially corn and soybeans, belong to a genetically modified variety (that is, they are genetically modified organisms or GMOs). Unfortunately, this way of feeding animals is completely different from the way animals were fed on family farms less than a century ago, and, consequently, these animals' digestive systems are not prepared to process these foods that are designed with the only purpose of fattening them. (Again, profits are maximized against the common interest.) Since feed pellets are not a natural food, the animals 1) live with chronic inflammation, which is the precursor condition for many diseases and 2) do not obtain the essential amino acids they would normally receive from their natural foods and have diets that are low in nutrients. Both of these circumstances make them prone to suffering acute gastrointestinal infections and other types of diseases, which is why they are administered antibiotics prophylactically.

In the case of poultry, to prevent parasitic diseases, increase their weight, and improve the pigmentation of their meat, there is a practice of adding a compound named Roxarsone to their food, which was used in the U.S. for over 70 years (and it continues to be used in other parts of the world). This compound contains an organic version of arsenic. Due to this method, the level of arsenic in poultry meat is three times higher than in any other meat. The problem with the organic version of arsenic is that, when the chicken is cooked, the element is altered to is inorganic version. Since antiquity, arsenic has been recognized as an extremely toxic chemical element that can produce nausea, vomiting, diarrhea, dehydration, and toxic shock. Long-term exposure has been associated with skin disorders, an increased risk of diabetes, high blood pressure, and different types of cancer. Inorganic arsenic has been considered a chemical cause of cancer.

The practice of adding arsenic to poultry bird feed began in the 1940s, but it wasn't until 2004 when a study for a scientific thesis drew consumers' attention. In 2009, the U.S. Food and Drug Administration (FDA) banned the practice of giving this type of supplement to poultry birds. In 2013, however, a group of farmers sued the FDA, and the process of removing this compound from the U.S. market was delayed until 2015. Unfortunately, the 70-plus years of exposure to this substance has had health consequences, and the practice is still allowed in many countries. You might be interested in knowing that the animal products with the highest amounts of organic arsenic are poultry and seafood (but in a form that is much less toxic than what's found in poultry).

๑๑ ๑๑ ๑๑ ๑๑ ๑๑ ๑๑

Intensive agriculture

Our modern society demands everything to be constantly productive. Unfortunately, this modern vision of efficiency exhausts our natural resources, land, air, and aquifers.

From the 1940s to the 1970s, the Green Revolution carried out studies, developments, and technology transfer initiatives. These practices increased food production around the world by developing high-yielding plant protein, expanding crop irrigation infrastructure, and distributing hybrid seeds, fertilizers, and synthetic pesticides to farmers. As cereals, grains, and legumes had become the main feed for farm animals, the increase in the supply of these foods cut the costs of animal products.

The industrial production of corn, soybeans, and wheat depends on synthetic fertilizers, herbicides, and pesticides, first, to artificially promote their growth and dominance over the other plant species they compete against and, second, to defend these crops from pests, insects, and other animal species. The problem with using synthetic fertilizers is that they are produced from a triad of nitrogen, phosphorous, and potassium (NPK). The lack of other minerals and compounds disturbs the underground ecosystem, impoverishes the land's biological activity, and causes a change in the composition of nutrients that the plants obtain from the substratum. Plants can survive on this cocktail of chemicals just as we can survive on "junk food," but it lowers their nutritional quality and leaves them vulnerable to pests and disease (which makes it necessary to use pesticides and herbicides with higher levels of toxicity). The USDA and the U.K. government have documented that crops treated with the chemicals in synthetic fertilizers, herbicides, and pesticides—since their introduction in the 1950s—have shown a considerable decrease in nutritional content, including vitamins A, B2 (riboflavin), C, and E, iron, calcium, zinc, selenium, and magnesium, to mention a few, along with certain phytochemicals (compounds that plants produce to defend themselves from pests and disease and that have antioxidant and anti-inflammatory effects on human begins).

What's more, there's some very bad news for industrial agriculture: It takes a few decades, at most, for competing weeds to grow resistant to herbicides and even less time for insects to develop immunity to pesticides. The bad news for us is that the agroindustry will continue to create even more potent and toxic herbicides and pesticides to counter the natural route of the species' evolution.

Intensive agriculture is centered on mono or dual crops (most are transgenic corn or soy). Monocrops, which cover vast areas, are not actually golden fields but rather extensions of land that have lost the diversity of species that would be naturally present in a balanced environment. These farming methods degrade the land as a result of the disproportionate use of water, fertilizers, herbicides, and pesticides. The reality is that these fields are biodiversity cemeteries because they displace other species and cause as much damage to ecosystems as industrial farms do. Over the past century, thousands of plant species have been pushed off the commercial chain because, driven by government subsidies, our farmers have opted to raise a handful of high-yielding[29] transgenic varieties whose harvesting and processing can be done mechanically.

---

[29] This refers to an efficient transformation of solar energy and soil minerals into macronutrients (carbohydrates, proteins, and fats).

It's also important for you to know that the genetic modifications these crops have been subjected to—the crops which, today, form the base of the products we consume—were not made to improve their nutritional content and benefit humanity but rather to improve the industry's profitability. In short, the main objective of genetic modification is to produce more calories per acre, even when the cost is the sacrifice of their vitamin and mineral content along with that of other essential compounds for human health. Once again, the industry has made its intention clear: to place the financial benefit of a few above the common good. Furthermore, this over-simplification of farming and harvesting processes has forced us to follow a diet with high concentrations of two dominant transgenic products: corn and soy.

Of the plant protein produced worldwide, 77% is used to feed animals on industrial farms, and the remaining 23% is mainly used to produce vegetable oils, sweeteners, processed foodstuffs, and cheap edible products with zero nutritional content. Junk food production is also part of the issue of environmental damage because it, too, promotes our disconnection with the Earth and its fruits. Because of this sea of misinformation and manipulation of knowledge that we are subjected to, it seems we've forgotten that human beings evolved as omnivores. This means that, in order to be healthy, we need hundreds of chemical compounds from a varied array of foods…not from two, or four, or ten…

Like the wise man from the story, Earth offers us all her fruits, but that's not enough for us nowadays. We prefer to exploit her. These intensive practices (in agriculture and livestock) are the result of our uncontrollable yearning for instant satisfaction (and the industry's insatiable desire for financial returns). Nothing seems to please us. Nothing seems to make us happy. We have also forgotten that sometimes "resting" is just as beneficial for animals, soils, plants, and the planet as it is for us. We all need to stop and take a breath now and then, including the Earth, because this is the natural process of life. But we have forgotten this because we rush through life, without stopping to observe or think, without pausing to see what's happening around us. In our frenzied lifestyles, we've forgotten that we depend on one another and that, by recognizing this interdependence and generously sharing the world with all its inhabitants (because there truly is enough for everyone), we'll have better opportunities for finding the happiness that we look for outside of ourselves with so much determination.

Remember, if we are not part of the solution, we're part of the problem. We must accept our share of the responsibility for the environmental deterioration that our generation is leaving behind to the planet. Don't you think it might be time to think about how to make this planet an equative and welcoming place for all of its inhabitants?

✂ 4 ✐

THE MYTHS WE'VE BEEN TOLD
SINCE WE WERE KIDS

THE BEST KEPT SECRET

I used to love the stories my grandmother would tell. She grew up in a small town in the Galician mountains and would tell me about how, when she was still very little, sometimes she would take the cows out to pasture. This activity was a bit scary for her and very tiring, and it took up a big part of the day. As she would walk away from the town, she'd start to feel afraid that some kind of animal might show up that would attack them, and so she would pray in order to feel calm. Because she was still just a girl, she used these outings as an opportunity to play with branches and stones, but she'd never lose sight of the herd. Each cow recognized my grandmother, and they all obeyed her when she announced that it was time to go home. They would walk back through the cloudy mountains and, as she hummed a tune, the cows would give her company.

In her town, they would celebrate the day when they killed a pig—traditionally during the coldest winter months—and they would use it from its tail to its ears. The party was meant to honor the pig and celebrate the food it provided. They would cure and salt the hams, shoulders, chorizo, bacon, sausages, and moronga, and then make morcilla sausages with the blood and save the rest in the lowest part of a cold shed. (This is why it was important to do it during the winter.) They would heat cauldrons over the fire to extract the fat and save it in large clay jars, and they would also smoke the blood sausages and other cuts of meat.

Since I didn't think the meat from just one pig would be enough to feed an entire family for a whole year, I asked, in awe, what they'd do when they ran out of food. She shrugged and, in a casual tone, answered that then they would just eat whatever there was. It's true that, since they had cows, her family used the milk to make cheese, curds, and curdled milk. They also had some hens, but the eggs, which were considered extremely valuable, were used for bartering; only on special occasions, such as to attend to an illness or during postpartum quarantines, did they eat eggs or make chicken broth. There was always rye or wheat bread on their table along with some of the vegetables that were a fundamental part of the Galician diet, such as potatoes, onions, garlic, cabbage, turnip greens, mushrooms, and peppers. There are also some legumes that grow in this region—haricot beans and chickpeas, for instance—and certain nuts, such as almonds, chestnuts, and acorns. They would season their food with spices such as bay leaf, oregano, parsley, paprika, and salt. And while they did have corn, they only used it to feed the pigs.

When she turned eight, my grandma left the mountains to move to the Port of Vigo, where her diet changed to be centered on mainly fish and seafood.

Now, if we were to base our analysis on our modern eating patterns (which claim that animal protein is the most important macronutrient, according to Liebig's theories), it might seem as if my grandma would have had nutritional deficiencies in the first years of her life, which are the most critical for human development. However, she was able to survive the ravages of the Spanish flu epidemic, the beginning of the Civil War, and moves from her town to Vigo and from Vigo to Mexico…and she lived a healthy life for over 90 years. She had the habit of going on long walks that many people half her age admired. Up until her last days, she was a strong woman who didn't show any signs of having suffered nutritional deficiencies in the first years of her life.

Proteins are fundamental organic molecules in our cells, and they are, indeed, the macronutrient that carries out most of the functions in our organism; they are necessary for forming tissues, enzymes, antibodies, and some neurotransmitters. So, are they important? Absolutely!

Proteins are made up of long chains of amino acids (which are their basic units) joined together by links called "peptide bonds," which form the protein structure. Science has identified 20 amino acids, but our bodies can produce only 11, which we call "non-essential." We know the remaining nine—that our bodies do not create—as "essential," and the only way to obtain them is through what we eat. These nine essential amino acids are lysine, methionine, threonine, tryptophan, valine, leucine, isoleucine, phenylalanine, and finally histidine, which is crucial in our early stages of life because children's bodies do not synthesize the required amount. The 11 non-essential amino acids are alanine, arginine, asparagine, aspartic acid, cysteine, glycine, glutamic acid, glutamine, proline, serine, and tyrosine.

Remember when I said that the talk about "including protein in our diets" is based on myth? What I meant is that dietary recommendations to "provide the body with the necessary proteins" actually refer to getting these nine amino acids from what we eat. What I've just said here is incredibly important because it's the clear explanation for why it doesn't make sense to talk about the quality of proteins in food. So, I'm going to repeat it…slowly:

The dietary recommendations to "provide the body with the necessary proteins"...

...actually refer to getting these nine amino acids...

...from what we eat.

After my second daughter was born, one of my aunts, whom I love dearly, recommended eating lots of meat because, as the popular saying goes: "*You need to eat meat to form muscles.*" So, I tasked myself with eating large helpings of animal products because I wouldn't spare any efforts to be healthy and strong to care for my baby. Lacking knowledge, I imagined that, upon entering my body, proteins would somehow be transferred directly to my muscles to fill empty spaces.

Now, I know the process is much more complex than that. From the moment we start chewing, two of the digestive system's most important functions begin: digestion and absorption. The process of digesting protein consists of breaking down peptide bonds to separate them into individual molecules, that is, into their basic units: amino acids. We could visualize amino acids as Tetris blocks (or, so younger generations will get what I'm talking about, Lego structures). After digestion, the absorption process is carried out to create our amino acid reserves. (This is something like sending the individual pieces— of whichever game you prefer—to be stored.) Later on, our bodies will use these individual molecules as needed.

Now comes a very important part, because you surely hadn't imagined that the human body *is* a protein factory and that our DNA holds the instructions for how to build these proteins. This is also very important, which is why I'll repeat it (not so slowly this time): the human body *is* a protein factory. They're not only necessary for forming muscles and tissues, but our bodies also need them to carry out many of its functions, including maintaining and regenerating cells, directing vital processes, regulating the expression of certain genes, and supporting homeostatic balance[30] (a self-regulation phenomenon that is in charge of an organism's internal maintenance). It should be clear to us that what this factory really needs in order to build proteins are the basic units, that is, the amino acids. The best kept secret is that our bodies do NOT need the chains of proteins as they are found in foods (long chains of amino acids joined together by peptide bonds) but rather the amino acids that the body stores during the absorption process (the individual "Tetris pieces" or "Lego bricks"). What's up to us is to supply our bodies with these nine essential amino acids—in whatever package they might come in. Are you following me?

When I replied that "I get my proteins from the same place that your proteins get theirs," what I meant was that grass—like all plants—is also made up of chains of amino acids. (Yes, any amino acid chain is a protein, so, grass has protein.) During digestion and absorption, a cow also breaks down the protein bonds and stores amino acids to, further along, build its new proteins according to its needs and unique biological processes. When we eat meat from a cow, our bodies break down the proteins that the cow had developed and recycle the essential amino acids that originally came from the grass it ate. The disadvantage of acquiring amino acids from cow meat is that they come with added saturated fats and toxins from the biological processes that living beings carry out in the simple act of living. Likewise, we bioaccumulate any chemical or synthetic compounds (such as antibiotics, hormones, pesticides, etc.) that the animal would have been exposed to along with any excess trace elements—iron, copper, zinc, or arsenic, to mention a few.

---

[30] From the Greek words *homo* and *estatis*, which mean "similar" and "stability," respectively.

So, where can we find the nine essential amino acids? It's true that these nine amino acids are found in foods of animal origin and that few foods of plant origin have all of them, but I bet no one ever told you that if we include a wide variety of legumes, whole grains, nuts, seeds, fruits, and vegetables in our diets, then there is no reason for us to have deficiencies since the amino acids that are missing in one variety (limiting amino acids) are found in another and vice versa. This is part of the magic of diversity and "protein complementation," which is the practice of mixing food families to get the nine essential amino acids.

For many years, animal products were cataloged as having high nutritional value for the sole reason of containing all the essential amino acids. Yet, today, research has acknowledged that, in addition to having proteins (despite being called incomplete), plants offer us other vital substances like vitamins, minerals, phytonutrients, antioxidants, polyphenols, water, glucose, and phytates, among other micronutrients that foods of animal origin do not provide. Science is starting to understand that the benefits these substances and compounds offer human beings make foods of plant origin an indispensable option for our long-term health. Flying the flag of "nutritionism," we've tried to isolate these substances, but we haven't gotten the expected results. Conclusions indicate a probability that obtaining benefits from each one of these elements is strongly related to the presence of other components in foods of plant origin. Moreover, it's been proven that isolating substances, like in the case of some antioxidants, is counterproductive. Even though foods of animal origin provide complete proteins, they are deficient in compounds that are essential for our health as well as fiber, which aids the passage through the digestive tract and feeds certain microorganisms that are vital for our health. A diet high in foods of animal origin also leads to an excess of saturated fats and toxins that our liver will have to remove. When we eat animal products, we increase the workload for this important organ, which, among other jobs, is in charge of processing fat as well as filtering and eliminating toxins.

In my grandma's experience, she had limited access to certain animal proteins during her childhood, but her diet also included legumes (fava beans and chickpeas), whole grains (rye and wheat bread), vegetables (potatoes, onions, garlic, cabbage, turnip greens, mushrooms, and peppers), nuts (almonds, chestnuts, and acorns) and spices. This combination provided her with the essential amino acids in times of scarcity and shortage. She got the nutrients that helped her grow up healthy and strong during the first eight years of her life and then until she reached the respectable age of 93. My grandmother's childhood could be used as an example of the effectiveness of protein complementation: Even though her diet was not predominantly based on animal protein for her first eight years, this did not generate developmental deficiencies. If you've been following me up until this point, the other good news, which you've surely already realized, is that you do not need to eat these nine essential amino acids in the same meal. Like I said earlier, your body stores them and, whenever your cells send the instructions to build new proteins, your body uses those stored amino acids according to its unique needs and requirements.

So, as long as you and your children try to eat a variety of food as part of a complete diet (avoiding cabbage or lettuce soup diets or anything similar), you shouldn't have any issues with your reserves containing the essential amino acids and your body having the supplies it needs to build this incredibly important macronutrient.

In the table next page, you'll find the food families and their limiting amino acids. The third column acts as a guide so you can get familiar with the food families that can be combined to ensure proper protein complementation:

Foods	Limiting Amino Acid	Complement with:
Whole grains (1)	Lysine and sometimes threonine. Corn is also deficient in tryptophan	Legumes, fruit, and vegetables
Legumes (2)	Methionine	Grains, nuts, and seeds
Nuts and Seeds (3)	Lysine and, in the case of almonds and macadamia nuts, methionine and tryptophan, respectively	Legumes, fruits, and vegetables
Fruits and Vegetables (4)	Methionine	Grains, nuts, and seeds

1) Whole grains: Grains are characterized by the seed and the fruit being one in the same. In contrast to processed grains, whole grains have three parts (the bran, endosperm, and germ). Examples: whole wheat, brown rice, wild rice, corn, barley, oatmeal, rye, sorghum, millet, teff, canary grass, quinoa, and amaranth.[31]

2) Legumes: These are the fruits of leguminous plants like lentils, chickpeas, fava beans, beans, soybeans, peas, and peanuts. Legumes have large amounts of lysine, threonine, and tryptophan.

3) Nuts and seeds: Nuts and seeds are energy-giving foods that are rich in fats and trace elements. Examples: walnuts, pecans,

---

[31] Quinoa and amaranth are known as pseudocereals because they actually belong to the same family as spinach, swiss chard, and beets.

almonds, cashews, macadamia nuts, hazelnuts, acorns, and pine nuts. Seeds could include pumpkin, sunflower, and sesame seeds (which is the seed that is richest in methionine).

4) Fruits and vegetables: Fruits contain at least one seed and develop from the flower of a plant, while vegetables consist of any other part of the plant such as stems, roots, leaves, bulbs, and flowers.

There are foods of plant origin that do have complete proteins, which I've listed below. To give you an idea of the equivalencies, every 3.5 ounces (100 grams) of meat have just less than 1 ounce (26 grams) of protein:

- Oyster mushrooms and some other mushrooms: a third of their weight is protein. Their water content is very high, which is why their caloric contribution is relatively low. They provide a considerable amount of fiber and vitamins B2 and B3. They're a good source of minerals such as selenium, potassium, and phosphorous and have bioactive components for treating and preventing different diseases, including regulating qualities of the immune system and blood sugar; hepatic protection; and anti-tumoral, antibacterial, antiviral, and antiparasitic properties.

- Quinoa: Every cup (185 grams) has 8 grams of protein in addition to being a good source of magnesium, iron, and zinc.

- Amaranth: Each cup (245 grams) has 9 grams of protein in addition to being an excellent source of magnesium, which is an important mineral for brain health. (It provides 100% of the daily requirement.)

- Chia seeds: Two tablespoons (28 grams) have 4 grams of protein, and they're also a good source of omega 3 fatty acids (which we'll talk about later on), calcium, iron, magnesium, and selenium.

- Spirulina: Every tablespoon of powder (7 grams) has 4 grams of protein, is rich in antioxidants, and is a good source of B complex vitamins, copper, and iron.

- Seeds or hemp hearts: Three tablespoons (30 grams) contain 10 grams of protein. They are particularly rich in essential fatty acids (omega 6 and omega 3) and are an excellent source of iron. They also contain phosphorous, magnesium, potassium, and zinc.

- Tofu, edamame, and tempeh: Each half cup of tofu and edamame (85 grams) contains 8 grams of protein, while tempeh has 11 grams. Tofu is an excellent source of calcium, and it also contains potassium and iron. Tempeh has fiber, iron, potassium, and calcium. Edamame also contains vitamin C.

Certain foods of plant origin have incomplete proteins of extremely high quality. If you properly complement the limiting amino acids of these foods, you'll get complete proteins with extraordinary properties:

- Beans: Each cup (240 grams) has 12 grams of protein.
- Lentils: Each half cup provides 9 grams of protein.
- Hummus (a creamy chickpea puree): 2 tablespoons (30 grams) have 7 grams of protein.
- Broccoli: Every cup contains 5 grams of protein.
- Peas: Each cup of cooked peas contains 8 grams of protein.
- Walnuts and pecans: 28 grams have an average of 6 grams of protein, but you should keep in mind that they have high caloric content.

The U.S. Recommended Dietary Allowance (RDA) for protein is 0.8 grams of protein for every kilogram of bodyweight, which equals 10% of the total daily calorie consumption; however, statistics show that in the U.S. the actual average consumption is around 16%. Now, let's review the percentage of protein we get as human beings from consuming our essential food: breast milk. It turns out that the portion of protein in breast milk, as a percentage of the total caloric content, is 5%. Isn't it strange that nature would decide, in the most critical moment of human development, that the proportion of the "master nutrient" would be half that of the RDA proportion or, for practical purposes, a third of the actual consumption shown in U.S. statistics? Protein plays a crucial role in mammals' growth and, as we've seen, it is also indispensable in all the processes that our bodies perform. Our current problem is not whether or not we consume protein, it's that our habits and customs have led us to consume it in excessive quantities. For most modern societies around the world that have access to exaggerated amounts of food and that, consequently, suffer overweight and obesity problems, wouldn't it seem that increasing the intake of protein is absolutely unnecessary?

The food industry built the current food system based on statements of an expert from the mid-19th century, losing sight of the benefits of food as a whole and magnifying the isolated properties of a macronutrient. While offering animal proteins at affordable prices was a solution for fighting malnutrition in the early 20th century, today, it makes us fall into excesses that are unleashing a global health crisis on a scale that has never been seen before. Once we've understood that our bodies actually need nine essential amino acids to build its own new proteins, saying that we need to get protein from food is as absurd as saying that we need to get blood or hormones in that same way too. All foods contain amino acids, which is why—in our day and age and in countries with a surplus supply of food—a protein deficiency is highly improbable. What we should be clear on is that the industry has taken advantage of the term—which is an isolated nutrient—to design, create, and construct an empire with the very specific aim of deceiving society so it can keep on with selling its products.

TIP #4: What can you do?

✓ While it may sound trite, it is fundamental that you and your children follow a balanced diet that makes room for fruits, vegetables, legumes, whole grains, nuts, and seeds.

✓ If you feel lost, look for support from your doctor, nutritionist, or an integrative health coach who is part of the pro-planet movement and knows how to combine the different types of foods.

✓ As an example, I'm going to tell you what a normal day is like for me, but I'll ask you to remember that every individual is unique and unrepeatable, and what works for my body might be counterproductive for someone else: After getting up, the first thing I drink is two cups of celery juice or, if I don't have celery, a glass of water with lime juice. A half hour later, I have a smoothy for breakfast that has fruit, vegetables, and some complete vegetable proteins such as amaranth, hemp, chia seeds, and/or spirulina. I make myself a half cup of coffee and then add oat milk. At noon, I eat carrots, jicama, or cucumber with lime, salt and chile and sometimes a handful of nuts with dates or a small portion of pumpkin seeds. On other days, I eat leftovers from the day before. For my main meal, I fix three dishes: an appetizer, an entree, and a side dish. I make sure the combination of these three dishes includes at least three food families (fruits and vegetables, whole grains, legumes, and nuts and seeds). I try to include a colorful salad and add pumpkin or sunflower seeds; as dressing, I just use a half teaspoon of olive oil, a pinch of salt, and a little fresh lime juice. For dessert, I eat a square of dark chocolate, maybe a piece of sesame brittle, and sometimes a bit of chili tamarind. In the evening, I generally eat three pieces of fruit, but sometimes I also eat a slice of toast (gluten free in my case) and spread peanut or almond butter on it. I also make thyme tea with fennel seeds and honey.

WE'RE NOT ALONE

"No creature is self-sufficient. Creatures exist only in dependence on each other, to complete each other, in the service of each other."

-Encyclical letter *Laudato Si'* of the Holy Father Francis
on the care of our common home

I really get a kick out of asking my clients if they know how many "human cells" there are for every ten cells that are found in the human body. I've gotten all kinds of different answers, from those who reply that all ten would have to be human to the most daring who, a bit unsure and in a curious tone, respond, "About five?"

The astounding answer is: "one." That's right, for every ten cells in the human body, only one is human. Breathe... Now that you've gotten past the shock, you'll surely want to ask, "And the rest?"

Let's go back in time some 4 billion years, several 100 million years after Earth was formed. The first life-forms on this planet were unicellular organisms that, over a remarkably long evolutionary process, started finding the way to interrelate with other organisms—which had different skills and qualities—to create synergies that made them more efficient or seek out associations to become larger organisms. Many microorganisms have preserved their original structure because they are crucial for supporting processes that allow life to exist on this planet. This is to say, microorganisms have existed forever; they are not invaders of our world as many people would like us to believe, and human beings have evolved for thousands of years, simultaneously establishing vital symbiotic relationships. Microbes found a protected habitat in human digestive tracts, with a stable temperature that also gave them a constant flow of nutrients. In exchange for this protection and controlled environment, they took charge of many processes related to digestion, nutrient absorption, and immunity. These organisms are better known as the microbiome or microbiota, and some reside in our skin, tissues, and mucus, but the vast majority are hosted in our intestines. For every ten cells in the human body, nine correspond to this type of organism, so—along the lines of what Deepak Chopra would say—we're a few human cells clinging onto a microbe colony.

The human body depends on these microorganisms so much that many of its processes are to enable them to flourish. For example, breast milk has three main components: lactose, fat, and certain types of carbohydrates known as human milk oligosaccharides (HMOs). What's interesting about this third majority, the HMOs, is that the human body is completely incapable of digesting them. So, why would the mother's body spend so much energy producing a substance that her baby can't digest or assimilate? The answer is fascinating. This important component of breast milk is a prebiotic; that is, a substance that feeds the microbiome. HMOs are specifically designed to nurture and encourage the dominance of the microorganisms that will be in charge of preparing the ideal conditions so a healthy microbiome can flourish in the baby's intestines: the *Bifidobacterium infantis*, also known as B-infantis. In short, HMOs are a compound that the mother's body produces for the sole purpose of feeding the microorganisms that are essential for the development of a healthy microbiome.

But what are the microbiome's functions? And what makes it important enough for a mother's body to invest the energy needed to produce these prebiotics in the milk that is exclusively designed to cover her baby's nutritional needs? Our digestive system is one of the ways we connect with the outside world, which is why it is fundamental for it to have a protective barrier against unknown substances or against those that could potentially be harmful for our organism. Some of the most important tasks of the microbiome are training cells from our immune system, protecting intestinal walls, and digesting and absorbing certain nutrients. The microbiome communicates with human cells and has direct access to the brain through specific hormones and the vagus nerve—something that modern science is starting to understand. As I mentioned earlier, the microbiome is made up of all kinds of microorganisms, and we have learned to work as a team with them. Certain viruses help us conserve the integrity of mucus and intestinal walls, other microbes form a line of defense against opportunistic or potentially harmful organisms, and several others carry out digestion and absorption processes that human beings are incapable of doing on our own (humans cannot digest fiber and certain types of sugars and fats).

There are also bacteria that are linked to the sensitivity of the vagus nerve's endings and others that are intimately related to producing hormones and neurotransmitters. For example, the microbiome produces over 90% of the serotonin in the human body. The processes that the digestive tract carries out are so important that some researchers have called it "the second brain." And it would seem that conditions like depression and other types of emotional imbalances have little to do with one's state of mind and are much closer related to an imbalance in the microbiome.

The training of our immune system is another one of the critical processes that these microorganisms carry out. Our immune system's job seems more like that of a forest ranger who wants to keep the ecosystem in balance. It has to pay attention to the type, quantity, and location of different colonies of microorganisms to ensure that the different species flourish in harmony…and it learns this from the microbiome.

What role do human beings play in this symbiotic relationship? Of course, we offer these microorganisms the convenience and comfort of our intestines, but we now have an even more important job—just as breast milk contains prebiotics for the first microbes to settle in our digestive system, it is our responsibility to continue to feed this microbiome with the proper nutrients. Obviously, this has just recently become our responsibility since our ancestors simply ate "food," and that took care of the matter. However, today, beyond food, we have a great variety of edible products and processed foodstuffs that offer zero benefit to our important guests and, in the worst of cases, starve them to death. This leaves the door wide open for pathogens and opportunistic organisms to settle into the gaps in our digestive system and create imbalances in our health.

Let me give you an example: If we don't eat fiber, we will lose the microorganisms that digest it, and if we lose them, then we'll get bloated whenever we eat fruits or vegetables. What I'm saying is that it's a vicious cycle. Then, we decide to take probiotics (which is another name for the microbiome), but they won't do anything for us if we aren't ready to feed them with the right foods. When we take probiotics, the most suitable thing to do would be to start eating the foods that make them flourish immediately (the next day). It's also important to pay attention to the strains of probiotics that we're taking—if the strain belongs to the *infantis* group, then you'll only be able to feed it by drinking breast milk. So, look for probiotics with a variety of strains and avoid those that only have strains from the *infantis* family. When you start taking them, immediately begin to eat foods that are high in fiber. Another way to keep your microbiome healthy is to plant your own herbs and spices (without herbicides, fertilizers, or pesticides) or to germinate some broccoli, alfalfa, clove, lentil, or sunflower sprouts at home. What's most important is to eat them without washing them first, since the layer of microbes that forms around the sprouts has the probiotics that are best for restoring the intestinal tract's flora. And so now you know that these modern times are forcing us to take responsibility for the foods we ingest in order to take care of our microbiome and keep it healthy.

We can also get an understanding of the importance of these microbes by approaching them from the viewpoint of the human genome. As human beings, we have around 25,000 genes that we receive in equal parts from Mom and Dad. While babies are in their mothers' wombs, these are the only genes their bodies have. When babies are born, ideally by passing through the birth canal, they acquire 2 million to 20 million additional genes. Yes, the moment of birth is when we are inoculated by our first microbiome, whose flourishing will heavily depend on the oligosaccharides from breast milk. So, the human genome forms a small part of the human being's genetic code, but it is mostly formed by the microbial genome, with an estimated ratio of 1 to 100.[32]

And so, we're not alone…

We already saw how diversity is one of the most important factors for maintaining the microbiome's health. Diversity is not only important in our internal ecosystem, but we now know that it is necessary to keep every kind of ecosystem balanced. We are not alone, and the evolutionary process has made us dependent on one another. The reality is that there are not good or bad microbes. What happens is that when things get out of balance and the conditions are ripe, one species will take advantage of the absence of another and colonize the empty spaces. However, when there's diversity, it's more difficult for an opportunistic species to colonize, first of all, because it won't find any room, but also because the other species will complement one another to protect this heterogeneity that offers space and opportunity to all.

Let's compare the microbiome with a figurative example: A fertile plot of land in the countryside will be open to the arrival of many species of animals, plants, and microorganisms. Each one of these species will benefit the others while also receiving its own gains. (In

---

[32] There are those who say this figure is very conservative and that the ratio is much higher.

symbiotic relationships, no one is anyone else's benefactor, and everyone complements one another as they search for their own benefit.) Dry leaves and organic compounds will serve as food for microorganisms, and they will provide plants' roots with crucial substances and components for their growth and defense against predators. Animals will eat the plants and their fruits and take on the task of spreading their seeds and spores throughout the field in their excrements. When they die, animals will turn into organic compounds and continue to nourish the land. The animals, plants, and microorganisms will live in a natural balance, and they will all receive from the ecosystem and also contribute to it.

But what would happen if we were to destroy the species living on this land and, in their place, plant vast fields of genetically modified corn? Naturally, other plants would start to appear and compete for nutrients, so farmers would spray the fields with glyphosate to kill the competing plants. The crops would be contaminated by this chemical, which would also harm the microbes and cause the soil to become increasingly more nutrient deficient. This situation would promote the use of synthetic fertilizers to artificially nourish the transgenic corn plants. The insects that might be interested in these plants will be exterminated with pesticides that will also kill some strains of microorganisms, making the soil lose microbial diversity. This will cause a sustained decrease in the soil's productivity until it becomes completely sterile. Since nature is wise, the plants sprayed with herbicides and the insects attacked with pesticides will start to build up resistance to these chemicals. They will become increasingly stronger, and only a handful of microorganisms will survive in the infertile soil. Along with the soil's productivity, the health of other plant and animal species will be put at risk, and the industry will be faced with the need to increase the toxicity of the fertilizers, herbicides, and pesticides. Sadly, the disruption of the land's natural balance will turn this field into a biodiversity graveyard.

Oops…it would seem that this isn't a hypothetical example…

What happened in this field is the same thing that's happening with our microbiome. We've changed the way we eat from following a varied diet rich in plant foods to a diet that basically consists of products from sick animals, junk food, and techno-foods (created from isolated nutrients or designed to be highly profitable). The saturated fat, toxins, chemicals, and synthetic components accumulated in these foods destroy part of our internal ecosystem's biodiversity and make way for invading and opportunistic species. Since this imbalance makes us sick, we turn to medicine and antibiotics that start to deplete the microbiome's ability to recover and carry out its critical functions that allow us to be healthy. Our intestines become increasingly more inhospitable, and this enables the preeminence of a handful opportunistic microorganisms. And then we resort to more potent medicine and antibiotics, leaving what was once a place brimming with life and diversity as a sterile terrain with only a few colonizing species that have claimed dominion.

The microbiome is very adaptable, and the composition of its internal ecosystem is unique. The way your microbiome is configured is closely related to the microbiomes of the people you regularly spend time with and to those of your pets. It depends on the place you were born, the place where you live, your cultural heritage and traditions, your medical background, and, of course, the way you eat. A diet rich in vegetables will create a composition that is very different from a diet rich in animal fat, and a change in diet (for example, from a local or traditional one to the standard American one) can unleash significant disruptions.

Likewise, we should remember that the toxic substances we ingest also affect the microbiome's composition. No one can deny the importance and effectiveness of antibiotics when it comes to fighting off certain infections that put our lives at risk, but we should know that—when we take them—they also wipe out part of our microbiome. While they have played an incredibly important role in treating many diseases and have saved countless lives, the abuse of antibiotics is turning them into a significant public health problem. Remember how farm animals are given antibiotics prophylactically to prevent disease? Now, I'm going to tell you about one of the theories of the effects of bioaccumulation, but first, it's important for you to know that there are two main reasons to perform genetic engineering on crops: 1) In order to make them resistant to herbicides, a gene from the *Agrobacterium* sp. strain CP4 bacterium—a microbe that is found in environments that are highly contaminated by glyphosate—is inserted into the plant's DNA (corn, soy, cotton, and canola, among others). 2) In order to make crops produce their own pesticide, a gene of the bacteria *Bacillus thuringiensis* is inserted into the plant's DNA (mainly corn and cotton), which produces a protein that is toxic for certain types of insects.

Well, here's one of the theories of the effects of bioaccumulation: These animals are fed cereals, legumes, and grains that were genetically modified, which were sprayed with herbicides (to eliminate the competing weeds) and pesticides (to prevent pests) and whose soils were bathed in synthetic fertilizers (to make up for the nutritional deficit). Cows eat the genetically modified plant protein (which includes one or both genes of the bacteria *Agrobacterium* sp. strain CP4, *Bacillus thuringiensis,* and diverse toxic substances derived from herbicides, pesticides, and fertilizers) and, in addition, they receive heavy amounts of antibiotics to prevent diseases like gastrointestinal infections, which are quite common. As human beings, when we eat their meat or by-products, we ingest the modified gene of one bacterium (or two)—which, according to the industry, does not affect the human genome, but whose effects on the microbial genome are still unknown. We bioaccumulate the toxic substances derived from the herbicides, pesticides, and fertilizers used on the crops, plus the antibiotics that they were given throughout their entire lives. Even though it still hasn't been scientifically proven, wouldn't it make sense to assume that eating an excess of these products might create an imbalance in our intestinal flora?

It is important for us to know and recognize that our health depends on other organisms. We are not alone, everything is connected, and in order to be well, both physically and emotionally, we should offer the best care and food to our incredibly valuable guests. I like to think about it in the same way Dr. Emeran Mayer portrays it in his book *The Mind-Gut Connection: How the Hidden Conversation Within Our Bodies Impacts Our Mood, Our Choices, and Our Overall Health*. He creates a beautiful metaphor, perfectly describing our microbiome as an intestinal orchestra made up of expert musicians who are ready to perform from the very first moments of our lives. The diets we choose not only determine what piece they'll play but also the quality of their performance. And our role? Well, we are the symphony conductors, and this is why taking care of our microbiome is so important.

TIP #5: What can you do?

- ✓ Take probiotics and try to switch brands throughout the year in order to include different strains. (Check to see that they have at least five strains and, preferably, that these strains do not belong to the *infantis* family.)

- ✓ Germinate sprouts of plants such as broccoli and radishes and add them to your salads without washing them. If you eat organic products and you know where they come from (your garden, your potted plants, a neighboring farm), don't wash them—just rinse them a little with water.

- ✓ You can consume fermented products such as miso, kombucha, coconut milk kefir, and fermented pickles (not vinegar pickles). While they can help with certain digestive problems, the microorganisms in these products multiply due to a decomposing process. Give preference to microorganisms that grow on living products (like those I mentioned in the first points).

✓ Buy organic fruits and vegetables, especially those from the Environmental Working Group's (EWG)[33] "dirty dozen" list because the pesticide content in their non-organic versions is very high (in 2021 the list included strawberries; spinach; kale, collard and mustard greens; nectarines; apples; grapes; cherries; peaches; pears; bell and hot peppers; celery; and tomatoes).

✓ Eat foods with high fiber content and avoid genetically and chemically modified foods.

✓ To the extent that is possible, and if conditions allow for it, avoid cleaning products that contain chlorine.

✓ Do not use insecticides inside or outside of your home.

✓ If you have pets, hug them and cuddle with them often and let your children do the same. Remember, the composition and health of our microbiomes also depend on the microbiome of the animals we spend time with.

---

[33] https://www.ewg.org/foodnews/dirty-dozen.php

INNOVATIVE RESEARCH

Throughout this book, we've seen that while the surplus supply of foods based on macronutrients (proteins, carbohydrates, and fats) does offer us short-term survival, the deficit in micronutrients can be a long-term threat to our health and our children's health. And this happens because when we focus on foods whose aim is to satiate our hunger—that is, foods that are rich in protein, carbohydrates, and fat—we take other foods off our plates that naturally contain vitamins, minerals, antioxidants, phytonutrients, and fiber, among others. Health results from a delicate balance between macro and micronutrients and, with the trend of nutritionism in full swing, we've forgotten that the best micronutrients are those that nature provides for us in their original packaging. Below, I'll present three relatively recent studies that explain some of the imbalances that originate from an excess—or deficit—of certain compounds in the human body. These imbalances are the result of the industrialization of foods and the processes that edible products are subjected to before reaching our tables.

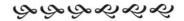

Iron

Aggregates known in the medical field as "amyloid plaques" have been found in the brains of people with Alzheimer's disease. They're formed by strands of beta-amyloid proteins and traces of aluminum, zinc, copper, and iron. Aluminum is definitely a compound that has no reason to be in our bodies, but we've accumulated it as a result of practices that simplify our daily lives (from cooking utensils, canned products, medicines, vaccines, etc.). However, zinc, copper, and iron are essential components, and they participate in some of the body's vital functions such as forming red blood cells and maintaining the health of blood vessels, nerves, the immune system, and bones. But zinc, copper, and iron are only useful for our bodies in exact quantities, that is, the excess of these compounds is toxic and can be counterproductive to our health (just as these amyloid plaques have confirmed). Iron and copper are highly unstable metals that can set off the production of free radicals (hydroxy, -OH), which causes oxidative stress in the body (inflammation), possible brain damage, and the acceleration of the aging process.

Our bodies use iron to produce hemoglobin, which is the protein that transports oxygen from the lungs to the rest of the body, and myoglobin, which transports oxygen to the muscles. Iron is essential for carrying out functions such as the production of oxidative energy, mitochondrial breathing, and DNA synthesis. Our bodies need iron to create hormones and connective tissues. When the amount of iron in the body shows a deficit, this causes a condition known as anemia. However, high concentrations of iron cause a condition known as hemochromatosis. Both alterations in iron content are harmful to our health.

Among the numerous false beliefs that I've been telling you about, there is also the assumption that foods of animal origin are the only ones that can provide us with the iron needed to carry out important functions. Let me explain what some doctors say, including Dr. Neal Barnard. Foods of plant origin contain iron known as "non-heme," while foods of animal origin contain small amounts of this type of iron but higher concentrations of what is known as "heme." For a long time, there was a belief that the human body absorbed "heme" iron better and that, to have the minimum required levels of this trace element, a much higher dose of the "non-heme" version would be necessary. For this same reason, it's common to think that animal products offer us a proper dose of iron while we would need an excess of products of plant origin to reach the minimum required intake.

However, recent studies have shifted this theory. The thing is that "heme" iron is more absorbable, but like everything in life, more doesn't mean better. Remember, the human body needs a specific amount. It's very hard for our bodies to regulate the absorption of "heme" iron, and even if our organism already has high concentrations, it will assimilate a large part of the iron contained in animal products. This happens because we bioaccumulate the iron that animals get from their food. Remember how we analyzed the consequences of bioaccumulation in previous chapters? In contrast, "non-heme" iron works in harmony with our organism: the body absorbs only what it needs and gets rid of the rest. That's why it might seem as if we absorb lower quantities, but it's actually a type of iron that works in a much smarter way, and our bodies take only what they need.[34] Plant-based foods balance iron in the body because plants have phytates that inhibit the production of hydroxyl free radicals and remove excessive iron through a process known as chelation.[35]

If we don't include plant-based products in our diet, the only way human beings can eliminate iron from the body is through menstruation or some other time of blood loss (like donating blood). Therefore, excessive iron in our diets is a risk. The amount of available iron has increased by one-third since the 1970s as a result of the fortification processes of edible products and processed foodstuffs. Deaths from hemochromatosis (according to death certificates) have increased by 60% (even though there's a belief that this number may be higher due to the fact that this condition is generally misdiagnosed).[36] It's important for you to know that, in addition to the

---

[34] Neal D. Barnard, MD, *Power Foods for the Brain: An Effective 3-Step Plan to Protect Your Mind and Strengthen Your Memory,* 2013.
[35] http://nutritionfacts.org
[36] Marion Nestle, *Food Politics: How the Food Industry Influences Nutrition and Health,* 2010.

iron contained in animal products, multivitamins and fortified foods (boxed cereals, bread, crackers, cookies, milks, etc.) contribute to an overdose of this trace element.

We all know that a lack of iron causes anemia and that this is a prevalent condition in cases of malnutrition. However, current rates of anemia in societies with high food supplies are very low (except in low-income communities and women of reproductive age). The reality is that between our current intake of food and edible products and the way we eat them, we are more likely to expose ourselves to an overdose of iron than to a deficiency. In addition to the most evident symptoms of intoxication from iron excess (fatigue, weakness, and pain) hemochromatosis is related to cardiovascular diseases, diabetes, liver damage, and arthritis, among others. In addition, and as I mentioned at the beginning of this chapter, recent studies about amyloid plaques conclude that excess iron can end up in our brains, causing various diseases that, today, are attributed to aging, but are actually directly related to our lifestyles.

That is, science is beginning to understand that diseases affecting the brains of people of advanced age start to take shape many years before signs of the condition show. Just as genetic disposition is an important component of diseases associated with cognitive skills (although today it is known that genetics is not destiny), everything seems to indicate that this is also true of high concentrations of certain compounds that we get through the foods we eat (specifically iron in this case).

ৎ৹ ৎ৹ ৎ৹ ৵৹ ৵৹ ৵৹

Vitamin B12

Vitamin B12 is vital for the health of the circulatory system and the central nervous system. A deficiency in this important vitamin has serious consequences, among which we can mention fatigue, weakness, pernicious anemia, shortness of breath, palpitations, visual difficulties, tingling in the hands and feet, lack of balance, memory loss, mental confusion, dementia, lack of appetite, mouth and tongue sores, and irritability. In addition, together with vitamin B6 and folate (also known as vitamin B9), it helps eliminate homocysteine from the body. Homocysteine is a small molecule that circulates through the bloodstream and originates as a temporary by-product when our cells build proteins. Homocysteine accumulates when there is a deficiency of vitamins B6, B9, or B12, and it has been tied to the risk of suffering heart attacks and strokes.

There is another false belief that has heavily permeated society that says people who consume animal products are not at risk of developing a vitamin B12 deficiency. It's true that neither plants nor animals produce vitamin B12; it is produced by a type of bacteria in the ileum, which is the last section of our small intestine. Considering that animals raised on industrial farms do not eat their natural foods (grass and foliage) but rather a mixture of genetically modified cereals, legumes, and grains (feed pellets), they also suffer nutritional deficiencies, including that of vitamin B12. What I'm trying to say is that you shouldn't get hung up on the misconception that consuming meat, eggs, or dairy products will provide us with the vitamins we need as human beings.

Unless you eat products from animals that lived in natural conditions (animals that graze freely in pastures), it's highly probable that your vitamin B12 levels are deficient. Don't think you're covered because you eat meat or products from industrialized animals. It's really important to keep an eye on your vitamin B12 levels so they don't become insufficient. In our modern times, all of us should take a supplement of this important vitamin.

TIP #6: What can you do?

✓ Eat products from free-range animals.

✓ Take a high-quality vitamin B12 supplement.

✓ As I recommended several chapters ago, plant your own herbs and spices (without herbicides, fertilizers, or pesticides) or germinate sprouts of plants such as broccoli, alfalfa, clove, lentils, or sunflowers at home and eat them unwashed. Along with its probiotics, the layer of microbes that forms around these foods also contains the type of bacteria that produces vitamin B12.

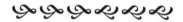

Essential fatty acids

Fats are key for our bodies to function properly. For example, they create energy reserves; protect our internal organs; are precursors for some substances; absorb vitamins A, D, E, and K; and are indispensable for building cellular membranes. In cellular membranes, fat forms a central layer and proteins adhere to it on both sides—we could imagine them as the filling of a protein sandwich made by these membranes. The type of fat affects the cell's general state of health along with its permeability, which is what allows for an exchange of compounds (such as glucose) to and from the exterior and vice versa.

But how do we know what the "good" fats are? These fats have been named fatty acids. The human body is capable of producing almost all of them, except those that are known as essential fatty acids. As you'll remember, the word *essential* is used to refer to substances and compounds that our bodies cannot produce, which is why we should get them through the foods we consume. Our bodies cannot produce certain omega 3 and omega 6 fatty acids, which are precursors of substances that regulate blood pressure, inflammatory and anti-inflammatory responses, and anticoagulant function, among others.

Omega 3 Fatty Acids

Healthy levels of omega 3 fatty acids have been tied to the reduction of LDL (low-density lipoproteins) cholesterol and triglyceride levels as well as decreased symptoms of cardiovascular diseases, diabetes, cerebrovascular accidents, rheumatoid arthritis, asthma, irritable bowel syndrome, ulcerative colitis, certain types of cancer, and mental disorders. In contrast, high levels of LDL cholesterol contribute to the accumulation of fatty acids in arteries and cause lesions in vascular walls, which reduces the diameter of the artery and blocks blood flow.

All food families of plant origin (fruits, vegetables, legumes, whole grains, nuts, and seeds) but especially seaweed (nori, spirulina, kombu, dulse, wakame, chlorella), leafy green vegetables (kale, spinach, purslane, brussels sprouts), and some nuts and seeds (walnuts, chia seeds, hemp, and flaxseed) contain traces of the omega 3 essential fatty acid "alpha-linolenic acid" (ALA). When we ingest ALA, it enters our bloodstream and, with the help of certain enzymes (these will be important later on, so don't forget about them), it is synthesized into two other omega 3 fatty acids: 1) eicosatetraenoic acid (EPA) and 2) docosahexaenoic acid (DHA).[37] To summarize, the three main omega 3 fatty acids are ALA, EPA, and DHA. (There are also other omega 3 fatty acids that are not considered essential such as HTA, SDA, ETE, ETA, HPA, and DPA, to mention a few.)

We can find ALA in all the food families and, with the help of certain enzymes (don't forget about them), our bodies synthesize EPA and DHA, which are essential for our brains: DHA influences the

---

[37] Chemically speaking, the 18 carbons of the ALA molecular chains extend to 20 carbons to form EPA and to 22 carbons to form DHA.

speed and quality of electric impulses between neurons, and it is a structural component of the skin and retina. EPA produces some molecules called "eicosanoids" that help us control certain mental functions and reduce inflammation. It's known that many modern diseases originate from a state of chronic inflammation that could be prevented by adequate EPA levels.

When ALA does not turn into EPA or DHA, the body simply stores it and uses it like any other fat. Many people claim that the best way to provide our bodies with EPA and DHA is through certain foods of animal origin, like fatty fish (salmon, tuna, sardines, mackerel, and trout) along with meat and dairy products, because the process of converting ALA to EPA and DHA is considered to be inefficient in the human body. On average, just one small portion of ALA turns into EPA (between 1% and 10%) and DHA (from 0.5% to 5%), and this conversion rate depends on trace elements and micronutrients such as copper, calcium, magnesium, zinc, and iron as well as vitamins such as B6 and B7. However, recent studies have determined that what is really happening is that enzymes that synthesize ALA (the ones I've asked you not to forget about) are used in other tasks that I will explain a bit later on.

Omega 6 Fatty Acids

Omega 6 fatty acids are also important for our health because they provide the building blocks for certain chemicals that are involved in the inflammatory response. This is incredibly important during the containment and healing processes of certain conditions that should be temporary, such as infections and lesions. Inflammation becomes a problem when this inflammatory process continues for prolonged periods because it starts to affect our health chronically. While it is a mechanism that the body uses to heal, when inflammation is an ongoing condition, it slowly affects our long-term health.

The most common omega 6 essential acid is "linoleic acid" (LA), and we get it from eating nuts, seeds, vegetable oils, meat, and dairy products. Omega 6 fatty acids are more stable than omega 3 fatty acids, which tend to spoil faster (they go rancid) and, therefore, processed foods have only omega 6 acids. Ideally, we should consume similar amounts of ALA (omega 3) and LA (omega 6), but LA levels have shot up in our modern diets due to the high consumption of vegetable oils, animal products, and processed products (with an estimated ratio of 17:1). Recent research indicates that this imbalance is a key component of the epidemic of chronic diseases that result from sustained inflammatory processes.

Now, I'd like to ask you to remember the enzymes I told you about a few paragraphs ago... Our bodies also convert LA into other omega 6 fatty acids according to their needs, and to carry out this process, they need the same enzymes that are used to convert ALA into EPA and DHA. The real problem is, since our modern diet has an excess in LA (remember the 17 to 1 ratio), the possibility of converting ALA into DHA and EPA is critically reduced. The imbalance created in our bodies by a high intake of omega 6 fatty acids led to the hypothesis that the human body lacks the ability to efficiently turn the omega 3 fatty acid ALA into EPA and DHA. The good news is that if we balance our consumption of omega 3 and 6, we can produce the proper amounts of EPA and DHA without needing to eat foods of animal origin.

You might be interested in knowing that studies have been conducted in Europe which conclude that the direct consumption of EPA and DHA (generally through fish-derived supplements) does not result in any improvement in different cognitive skills if these supplements are not accompanied by a reduction of omega 6 fatty acids.

Also, remember that the term bioaccumulation was initially coined to explain the accumulative effects of toxic components on the marine food chain. When we eat large fish with a high fat content, such as tuna or mackerel, not only are we obtaining omega 3 fatty acids, but we are also bioaccumulating substances and compounds that are toxic for the brain, such as mercury (methylmercury) and other contaminants that they have obtained from their food. It's also important for you to know that only between 15% and 30% of the fat from fish is equivalent to omega 3 fatty acids; the rest, from 70% to 85%, is a mixture of saturated, monounsaturated, and polyunsaturated fats. Not that I want to disappoint you even further, but fish also contain cholesterol, and some seafood, like shrimp and lobster, have more cholesterol than red meat. Another thing I want to share with you is that marine animals get their omega 3 fatty acids from seaweed and algae, so you can skip the intermediary and go directly to the source without any issue.

TIP #7: What can you do?

✓ Complement your meals with seaweed and leafy green vegetables as well as chia seeds, hemp, and flaxseeds.

✓ Since omega 3 fatty acids go rancid quickly, keep your chia seeds, hemp, and flaxseeds in the refrigerator.

✓ Decrease the use of cooking oils to a minimum, using only what's necessary.

✓ Significantly reduce your consumption of processed foods. Remember, they are all made with omega 6 fatty acids, and we want to find a balance between omega 3 and 6.

✓ Reduce (ideally, avoid) protein from animals that were fed pellets.

✌ 5 ✎

THINGS TO KEEP IN MIND

SOME NOT-SO-FUN HORROR STORIES

Accoring to the World Health Organization (WHO), chronic diseases—also called lifestyle diseases—are the greatest cause of death worldwide, and this figure by far surpasses cases of death due to infectious and contagious diseases. Heart diseases together with strokes and chronic obstructive pulmonary disease account for 33% of these deaths (18.4 million in 2019).[38]

Obesity is a chronic disease that takes around 2.8 million lives each year and is cataloged as a form of malnutrition on the 2030 Agenda for Sustainable Development, whose goal is not to "eradicate hunger" but to ensure people's "access to sufficient and nutritious food." The obesity pandemic has become one of the primary public health issues. This means that obesity and its consequences are a major socioeconomic problem worldwide. Moreover, even while obesity is recognized as a global crisis, it's important for you to know that, paradoxically, the UN reports more than 1 billion people around the

---

[38] https://www.who.int/news-room/fact-sheets/detail/the-top-10-causes-of-death

world are living with hunger.[39] In the U.S., treatment for chronic diseases costs nearly $150 billion a year—a figure that continues to grow—and one in every five children along with one in every three adults is overweight or obese.[40] Because of this pandemic, in my home country of Mexico, for example, we are on the verge of a public health crisis (it's estimated that in 2030, 40% of adults will be obese). What's more, according to the Organisation for Economic Co-operation and Development (OECD), it's the country with the second highest percentage of out-of-pocket health expenses,[41] "out-of-pocket expenses" referring to the costs that families allocate directly to covering different health care requirements (not including private health insurance).

But why are we obese?

As we've seen, fats are necessary for the proper functioning of our bodies. But not all fats are the same, and some are better than others. The fats in animal products are saturated fats, and the problem with this type of fat is that they alter blood lipids. Saturated fats cause 1) an increase in total cholesterol and LDL and 2) a decrease in HDL (high-density lipoproteins, which transport the cholesterol from all our tissues to the liver so this vital organ can eliminate it), and this combination sets off the risk of suffering cardiovascular diseases. Likewise, it has been proven that the excessive consumption of these fats causes chronic inflammation in the digestive system, which quickly replicates throughout the rest of the body.

Let's go over what happens in our bodies when we live with chronic inflammation. The hypothalamus is the gland that regulates our needs for ingesting food, and it receives information from the

---

[39] Food and Agriculture Organization of the United Nations, "The State of Food Security and Nutrition in the World," 2019.

[40] Department of Health and Human Services, Center for Disease Control and Prevention, "Overweight and Obesity."

[41] IMCO Staff, Instituto Mexicano para la Competitividad, "Pequeños pasos para transformar el sistema de salud."

digestive system through 1) the hormones in charge of activating or deactivating the appetite that travel to this gland through the bloodstream and 2) the vagus nerve's satiety sensors. The vagus nerve has endings in the throat, lungs, heart, and digestive organs, and, accordingly, it is known as a "pneumogastric nerve." This nerve controls respiratory rhythm, strength, and frequency, and it works in a circuit: it sends messages from the brain to the organs and vice versa. It is through these messages that the body prepares for the fight or flight response. Because these sensors are responsible for the satiety response, when there is a state of chronic inflammation that blocks sensors from the vagus nerve, our capacity to sense when we have eaten enough is reduced. What we know now is that eating in excess does not come from a lack of willpower: it results from the chronic inflammation of nerves due to an exaggerated intake of saturated fats of animal origin.

And cholesterol?

Some studies conclude that an excess of cholesterol in the blood and its deposits in arteries represent one of the risk factors for cardiovascular diseases. However, in the literature, you can find the lipid hypothesis—established in the 1950s—which has observed a direct relationship between mortality from coronary diseases and the consumption of saturated fats. It's still under debate. The liver produces 75% of the cholesterol found in the human body because the body needs it to form substances such as vitamin D, hormones, and bile acids, and we get the remaining 25%, primarily, from the animal products we consume. Recent studies have discovered that saturated fat stimulates the liver to produce cholesterol. That is, animal products give us double the cholesterol: what's in the food plus what our liver makes when stimulated from its saturated fat content.

What food has the highest fat content?

Unfortunately, "nature's" so-called "perfect food" (along with its by-products) is the animal product with the highest saturated fat content. Just to give you an idea of the amount of fat contained in dairy products, I'll list the proportion of fat as a percentage of the caloric content of these different foods: butter 100%, various types of cream 97%, American cheese and cream cheese 74%, ice cream and whole milk 48%, cottage cheese 38%, and low-fat milk 34%. So, if you've heard that drinking milk helps you lose weight, ask yourself if this is not yet another myth created by the industry and backed by organizations such as the US National Dairy Council (NDC), which upholds that consuming dairy products is tied to improved bone health, lower risks of developing type II diabetes, and a decrease in cardiovascular diseases.[42] Based on the Dietary Reference Intakes (DRIs), the NDC recommends consuming three servings of dairy each day. DRI is the general term for a set of reference values used to plan and assess nutrient intakes of healthy people. In the 1990s, as a measure for fighting hypertension caused by excessive sodium in the standard American diet (SAD), the DRI for potassium ingestion was doubled. Dairy products contain potassium, which is why, in order to meet this new DRI, nutrition recommendations for consuming these products increased from two to three servings a day. The problem is, while dairy products do contain potassium, they also contain sodium and saturated fats. What's interesting here is the reasons why the Advisory Committee (which is in charge of defining nutrition guidelines and recommendations) established that potassium requirements would be met through an increase in the consumption of dairy products, considering that fruit and vegetables also contain potassium and do not produce negative effects like those from the sodium and saturated fats from dairy. At this stage in the game, and with everything I've been telling you about, this should come as no

---

[42] https://www.nationaldairycouncil.org/health-and-wellness

surprise: the Advisory Committee was made up of eleven individuals, seven of whom were heavily involved in the industry.

In addition, there's another important issue we should consider when speaking about dairy products: their powerful addictive effects. Let's take it step by step. We shouldn't be surprised by the fact that milk—from any mammal—has addictive substances. Nature is wise, and this is how it ensures babies will return to their mothers to get the nutrients they need to grow, while the mother and her offspring also develop their corresponding affective bonds. Casein is a protein with narcotic qualities that is found in cow's milk, and it is the source of the compounds known as exorphins (casomorphins). Remember that when proteins are digested, they are broken down into their basic units that we know as amino acids. Well, proteins are not always completely broken down, and, sometimes, a few amino acids stay joined together (as if they were smaller protein chains). These compounds are known as peptides. Exorphins are opioid peptides (they're called opioids because they join together with opioid receptors that are located in the central nervous system and the gastrointestinal tract), which are produced when gluten and casein proteins are digested. It's believed that gluten and casein form peptides (instead of breaking down into amino acids) because their peptide bonds are resistant to certain enzymes in the digestive process. These exorphins have pain regulation qualities (they release dopamine), but they also cause addiction. In cheese, casein is eight times more abundant than it is in milk because of the reduced amount of water, lactose, and whey, which makes it a powerfully addictive product because it gives the body a higher dose of casomorphins. There is no animal product more addictive than cheese.

While we're at it, why don't we just keep throwing fuel on the fire… Milk is, by nature, a hormonal product. In it, you can find hormones from certain glands, like the pituitary gland, thyroid, and hypothalamus, as well as estrogens, progesterone, IGF-1[43] (a natural hormone that stimulates cell division and activates the growth of mammary tissue during puberty; it diminishes as we age) and other growth factors. Additionally, in many places around the world (including the U.S. and numerous Latin American countries) it is legal to inject cows with a chemical hormone known as rBGH (Recombinant Bovine Growth Hormone), which is genetically designed to increase milk production. Its use started to be more commonplace in the late 1980s, but this practice has since been banned in the European Union, Australia, Canada, and Japan (the reason being that there are scientific studies proving rGBH to cause cancer in rats). It's been confirmed that when cows are injected with this chemical their IGF-1 levels increase. There still isn't scientific basis for this next statement, but if you have daughters under the age of 10 who have started developing mammary tissue, it might be a good idea for you to consider the possibility of eliminating cow milk from their diets.

Finally, the cherry on top... The consumption of dairy products has been linked to some common diseases in children, such as allergies, acne, anemia, constipation, colitis, eczema, gastrointestinal diseases, and ear infections. Furthermore, recent studies have discovered a correlation (remember that correlation does not imply causation) between consuming dairy products and certain ailments such as cardiovascular diseases, type I diabetes, autism, arthritis, sinusitis, leukemia, and lymphoma.[44] There are no conclusive reviews about the relationship between the consumption of dairy products and breast or prostate cancer, but there are isolated studies that determine that, upon eliminating dairy products, the tumors and cancer diminish or disappear entirely. It would seem, then, that nature's perfect food is, indeed, perfect for calves, but not so perfect for human beings.

---

[43] Insulin-like growth factor 1
[44] Joseph Koen, *Whitewash: The Disturbing Truth About Cow's Milk and Your Health*, New Society Publishers.

As I mentioned earlier, if you have questions about what I've just presented, review the sources, research who funded the studies you've seen, analyze who comes out the winner with the results that are presented, and remember that the industry will always have an argument or publicity stunt and will also offer you opinions from nutrition experts (whom they've confused in one way or another or who are financially dependent on the same industry). They'll do this to seductively invite you to keep consuming their products. Unfortunately, for many years, the food industry's conduct has had one sole aim: to satisfy its interests and its interests alone. This industry does not care about your health or well-being, and it doesn't care about your family's health and well-being either, or that of your community, or that of society at large, and much less about that of future generations. Don't forget the 40-year war against smoking tobacco, which the industry took advantage of to confuse the public while it kept raking in millions of dollars in profits. The food industry works the same way (you may not have realized that tobacco giants own the food companies…but they do), and its only purpose is to sell, sell, sell, and, therefore, maximize earnings, not in benefit of humanity, but rather in the favor of just a few.

ANCESTRAL WISDOM AND PREDICTIONS OF THE FUTURE

"If someone wishes for good health, one must first ask oneself if he is ready to do away with the reasons for his illness. Only then is it possible to help him."

-Hippocrates

The therapeutic approach to Hippocratic medicine is based on the curative power of nature. Despite the beliefs of his contemporaries, who were certain that illnesses were caused by falling from the grace of the gods,[45] Hippocrates offered a physical and rational explanation to describe their origin. First and foremost, he held the belief that the human body has the intrinsic power to recover and heal—as part of its natural processes—through a proper lifestyle. The lifestyle he promoted included: 1) a good diet, 2) adequate rest and recovery, and 3) cleanliness and a quality environment. His focus promoted what is known today as preventative medicine. A well-known phrase that is attributed to him is: "Illnesses do not come upon us out of the blue. They are developed from small daily sins against Nature. When enough sins have accumulated, illnesses will suddenly appear."

Some 500 years later, Seneca, an extraordinary speaker and tutor and advisor of the emperor Nero, wrote: "An Ox is satisfied with the pasture of an acre or two: one wood suffices for several Elephants. Man alone supports himself by the pillage of the whole earth and sea. What! Has Nature indeed given us so insatiable a stomach, while she has given us so insignificant bodies? No: it is not the hunger of our stomachs, but insatiable covetousness (ambitio) which costs so much. The slaves of the belly (as says Sallust) are to be counted in the number

---

[45] Hippocrates was born on the island of Kos, Greece, in the year 460 BCE

of the lower animals, not of men. Nay, not of them, but rather of the dead. ...You might inscribe on their doors, 'These have anticipated death.'"

For thousands of years, there have been diverse discussions on the source of health, the cause of illness, and the greed of human beings. *The Republic* by Plato, written around the year 390 BCE, covers the ideas of his philosophy and work in ten books that contain dialogues between Socrates and other philosophers of the time. The dialogue between Socrates and Glaucon (Plato's brother, a Greek philosopher, who appears as an interlocutor in *The Republic*) centers on the codes of the ideal State. As part of these codes, Socrates suggests a moderate diet that would offer the population a peaceful and healthy life, in harmony with the environment. Glaucon argued that the cities of the future would need a modern diet that could afford the luxury of eating meat. Socrates was known for his speaking skills and his use of irony to ridicule arguments that were contrary to his own. This tactic of his made his interlocutors fall into contradictions, and this is how he taught his disciples to reflect on their arguments and foster debate. Glaucon's response led Socrates to ask the following:

> Would this habit of eating animals not require that we slaughter animals that we knew as individuals, and in whose eyes we could gaze and see ourselves reflected, only a few hours before our meal?
>
> And, if we pursue this way of living, will we not have need to visit the doctor more often? *(Referring to the state of inflammation caused by consuming animal products, something that was already known in this era.)*
>
> If we pursue our habit of eating animals, and if our neighbor follows a similar path, will we not have the need to go to war against our neighbor to secure greater pasturage, because ours will not be enough to sustain us, and our neighbor will have a similar need to wage war on us for the same reason?
>
> Would not these facts prevent us from achieving happiness, and therefore the conditions necessary to the building of a just society, if we pursue a desire to eat animals?

The text explains that Glaucon assented to each of these questions, which forced him to change his opinion. In other words: Socrates used the maieutic method (a form of dialogue through which the interlocutor is questioned, discovering truths for him or herself) to demonstrate to Glaucon that by including animal products in a "luxurious" diet, modern cities would be tainted from taking the lives of innocent beings. They would be filled with disease, conditions, and ailments, and they would face war and violence over the possession of land because more territory is required to raise animals for human consumption...circumstances that were very different from the ideal state of happiness and justice. It would seem that Plato had known, even at that time, that feeding mainly on animals is not the key to health, prosperity, and happiness, and that—in addition to bringing illnesses to humanity—this false sensation of richness and luxury would cause the deterioration of the environment and society.

And these are precisely the challenges we are facing now...

I don't know what you think, but it seems to me that, in this day and age, we are experiencing humanity's worst ailments and seeing levels of destruction and devastation like never before. Perhaps it's time to reflect, as Hippocrates said, about whether our sins against nature have accumulated in excess and, as Seneca warned, if we are anticipating death.

Much later, in the early 19th century, two major schools of thought in medicine started debating about how to address illnesses. The first described illness as a result of an imbalance in the human body from an integrative or holistic viewpoint (very similar to Hippocratic thinking). The second upheld that illness was caused by the intervention of an external agent that affected a specific body part or organ. This discrepancy between medical approaches gave way to the struggle between the theories that understand illness as a holistic issue—and focus on improving and maintaining health through integrative nutrition and lifestyle—and those that see it as the result of isolated events which affect a specific organ or tissue and that should be fought with chemicals or medicine.

The school of thought that understands illness as a matter of isolated and localized conditions has driven the pharmaceutical industry's flourishing dominance. As a result of this industry's boom and the financial power it has gained over the years, a debate has begun in various forums about whether or not it is an ethical practice to allow those who are in charge of telling us how to be healthy to also be the ones who are providing us with the medicines and substances to reach this ideal health. That is, society has started to question the pharmaceutical industry's role of both judge and jury because, in addition to the fact that this combination of functions has made it a highly profitable industry, the vast majority of us have been left with no understanding of what lifestyle changes are really necessary to reach an optimal state of long-term health.

The school of thought that addresses health issues through diet is a two-sided coin. The first side is not so uplifting, given that, as in the case of the pharmaceutical industry, the companies that tell us what we should eat are the same ones that benefit from our eating habits. And here's where we're really trapped, because these companies have arranged and conditioned our behaviors through advertising campaigns that distort information (like the examples I've been mentioning throughout the book). However, the other side of the coin is more heartening: it's the recommendation to return to the food of the Earth, the food that grows because it is full of life and, consequently, offers us life. It's about reconsidering plants as a central part of our diets, because their nutrients come from the soil's biological activity, and they grow with energy from the sun.

To create economic wealth in the benefit of just a few, the food industry has plotted an infinite number of schemes to drive society to live in a pressing state of excess. This lifestyle is leading us to suffer illnesses caused by wealth and luxury and to lose sight of the repercussions of our decisions. For example, it takes approximately 2.6 pounds (1.2 kilograms) of plant protein to put the total daily recommended servings of meat on your table (7 ounces or 200 grams). This information gets even more interesting once you learn that these 2.6 pounds of plant protein could feed 24 people without issue. I would like to add that for every kilogram of animal protein produced, livestock is fed nearly 13 pounds (6 kilograms) of cereals, legumes and/or grains. Remember that, due to inequitable food distribution, over 1 billion people go to bed hungry each night, but the same number of people go to bed with overweight or obesity issues.

Never before has food been so cheap, but we're paying for these low costs with our health and the planet's health as well. We are starting to pay the true price, but it will be the future generations who actually end up paying for it. Children's health problems around the world are alarming: In the U.S., one in three children show early signs of heart-related illnesses. Up until a few years ago, type II diabetes, high blood pressure, and gallstones were considered diseases that exclusively affected adults, but now they also affect children and youth. Obesity has duplicated in children and tripled in adolescents; today, over 23 million children and adolescents in the U.S. are obese or suffer from being overweight. One in every seven young people is obese, and one in every three is overweight. According to certain estimates, this will be the first generation to live with more illnesses and die much younger than the generations of their parents and grandparents. Yet, this situation shouldn't only concern us as an isolated health issue: the consequences of obesity represent a threat to many countries' social security systems as well as to the global economy. Child obesity increases the risks of cardiovascular diseases, high cholesterol levels, asthma, cerebral infarctions, some types of cancer, and diabetes.

And these are the excesses, the need to satiate rather than nourish, that have led society to fall ill: obesity, overweight, digestive problems, loss of cognitive abilities, body pain, migraines, diabetes, cancer, and strokes, along with a whole array of mental illnesses and cardiovascular, respiratory, autoimmune, and chronic-degenerative diseases…and the list goes on.

Moreover, we have reached a point in history at which our systems of production, use, and consumption are not sustainable or justifiable. Never before has humanity been so destructive. We are ravaging our soils, aquifers, and forests; we are polluting the air we breathe and causing adverse changes to the atmospheric composition; and we have been exterminating plant and animal species at an unprecedented rate. The massive scale at which genetically modified plants have been introduced is devastating, and the environmental repercussions this abuse will have on the future are still unknown to us. When a part of the food chain is disrupted, it affects all the beings that depend on it. If the soil is diseased, that means it is deficient and that the plants growing in it will also be. This imbalance will also cause nutritional insufficiencies in the animals that feed on it. Therefore, human health is intimately related to the health of soil, water, and air, but also to the health of other beings, like microorganisms as well as larger animals. That is, our health and the planet's health cannot be addressed in an isolated manner. And while those who seek personal financial gain have led us to believe that this mass destruction is not our responsibility, it is urgent that we start to recognize the planet's current situation as a result of our lifestyles and the decisions we make about our next meal.

I don't want to sound "apocalyptic" (which was what my dad told me when he read the first draft of this book), but we have a situation here, and we must decide if we are going to fall into a collective state of disease, poverty, and degradation or if we will opt to make the changes that are necessary to improve our health and the planet's health. Our ancestors, who understood their relationship with the environment and the behavioral patterns of different social groups, sorrowfully envisioned one of the possible paths that humanity might take and, sadly, it is the one our generation has chosen. But not all is lost. I do believe there is hope. I believe we can still face what might seem irreparable and turn it around. I believe that each and every one of us is great and strong enough to contribute to this change.

To close this chapter, which has hopefully served as a useful reflection, I'll leave you with a few fragments from the fable of Chief Seattle of the Suquamish tribe in response to the white men who wished to purchase his people's land. While the letter is, in fact, a cinematic myth, its words of poetic wisdom still resonate:

> How can you buy or sell the sky—the warmth of the land? The idea is strange to us. [...] Every part of this Earth is sacred to my people. Every shining pine needle, every sandy shore, every mist in the dark woods, every clearing, and every humming insect is holy in the memory and experience of my people. [...] The scented flowers are our sisters: the horned beasts, the horse and the majestic eagle are our brothers. The fields, the warm body of the foal and man, all belong to the same family. [...]

> If we sell you these lands, you must remember that they are sacred, and teach your children that they are, and that every ghostly reflection in the clear waters of the lakes speaks of the lives and memories of the life of my people. The murmur of the stream is the voice of my father's father. [...]

> We know that the white man does not understand our ways. One portion of land is the same to him as the next, for he is a stranger who comes in the night and takes from the land whatever he needs. The Earth is not his brother, but his enemy, and when he has conquered it, he moves on. He leaves his father's graves and his children's birthright is forgotten. He strips the Earth from his children and cares not. [...]

> He treats his mother, the Earth, and his brother the heavens, as if they were things that could be bought, plundered, and sold, as though they were lambs and glass beads. His insatiable hunger will devour the Earth and leave behind a desert. [...]

The air is precious to the redman. For all things share the same breath—the beasts, the trees, and the man. The white man does not seem to notice the air he breathes. Like a man dying for many days, he is numb to the stench. If we sell you our lands, you must remember that the air is precious to us, that the air shares its spirit with all the life it sustains. And, if we sell you our lands, you must set them aside and keep them sacred as a place that even the white man may go to taste the wind sweetened by the flowers in the grasslands. [...]

If I decide to accept, I will make one condition. The white man must treat the beasts of this land as his brothers. [...] What is man without the beasts? If all the beasts were gone, men would die from great loneliness of spirit, for whatever happens to the beast also happens to the man. All things are connected. [...]

You must teach your children what we have taught ours: that the Earth is our mother. Everything that affects the Earth affects the sons of the Earth. When men spit on the ground, they spit on themselves. We know this: the Earth does not belong to man. Man belongs to the Earth. Man has not woven the net of life: he is just a thread in it. Everything he does to this net he does to himself. What befalls the Earth will befall the sons of the Earth. We know this. All things are bound up in each other like the blood that binds the family.

When the buffalo are all slaughtered, the wild horses all tamed, the secret corners of the forest heavy with the scent of many men, and the view of the ripe hills blotted by the talking wires, where is the thicket? Gone. Where is the eagle? Gone. And what is it to say goodbye to the swift and the hunt?

The end of living and the beginning of survival.

YOU CAN CHANGE THE WORLD

L et's get romantic and imagine an ideal world...

♥ Governments do the job they are actually supposed to do: protect citizens from the dishonest practices of corporations.

♥ Public policies include a new definition of the meaning of *food*, which is explained as the sustenance that should lead society to maintain optimal health in the long term. The definition clarifies that *food* refers to the provisions that come from the Earth and have been with human beings throughout an evolutionary process of thousands of years and are reaped in harmony with the planet, respecting a model of environmental circularity. Reincorporating the word *food* into laws displaces nutritional terms that have kept society confused for decades.

♥ Public health laws grant incentives to those who seek out better diets; for example, an organic apple is half the price (or less) of the cost of a bag of junk "food" (or a protein bar, which would be the same in this case).

♥ Government subsidies are used to put true food within reach of society.

♥ Laws establish that if the industry produces and/or sells harmful foodstuffs or edible products, not only will they not be subsidized, but they will also be sanctioned and come with a higher tax burden.

❤ Advertising expenses to promote foods are banned, and these resources are allocated to the common good, to restoring ecosystems, and to supporting marginalized communities.

❤ Public health laws are based on the population's health and environmental care. Their main objectives are balance and prevention.

❤ Both governments and corporations have a vision for the future surrounding health and environmental issues.

❤ The foundation of the agroindustry is made up of family and local farms. Their practices are sustainable and incorporate models of soil regeneration and environmental care, and they respect models of environmental circularity.

❤ The health system goes beyond treating illnesses and includes all spheres of life: physical, mental, emotional, social, and spiritual.

Now, let's get back to the (sad) reality…

✗ Over the past decades, the food industry has invested millions and millions of dollars—with backing from the government and experts—to see to it that we make the wrong decisions as consumers.

✗ The messages on the labels of industrialized products are deceiving, and corporations have taken advantage of the confusion of nutritionism to falsely state that their junk "food" is beneficial to our health.

✗ Subsidies and lobbying are another disadvantage for consumers; for example, in the U.S., subsidies for the meat and dairy industries amount to $38 billion a year, while the sum of subsidies for specialized foods (understood as fruits and vegetables) is only $17 billion. The meat industry makes multi-million-dollar contributions to political campaigns and then still contributes more to lobbying the federal government. According to varied analyses from the U.S. Department of Commerce of the change in the consumer price indexes, from 1980 to date, the indexed price of fruits and vegetables has increased by 40%. And to add insult to injury, in this same period, the indexed price of other products such as butter, beer, and soft drinks has dropped by 15% to 30%.[46]

✗ Agroindustry is a very important part of the world economy. In the U.S., the agricultural and livestock sectors are among the primary economic activities, representing 2% of the country's annual GDP. According to the American Meat Institute, this industry contributes $900 billion to the U.S. economy. Governments have their hands tied because the economy heavily depends on these corporations.

✗ Much of the information we receive from "nutrition experts," whose approach is solely focused on nutrients, is harmful to our health, to our children's health, and to the planet's health.

✗ Human health has been sacrificed before large corporations' thirst for profit, and there is no government, scientific group, or medical system that the industry has not compromised in one way or another. The restoration of our health is truly in our hands.

But let's not get too distraught…

It's quite likely that the more information you find about what is in the products you eat, where they come from, what's behind them, and how they are sold to you, the angrier, more frustrated, and more manipulated you'll feel. By now you're surely wondering how we can continue to have edible products within our reach and keep buying and eating them when we know they are harmful for our health, our

---

[46] Figures reported on the Center for Responsive Politics' OpenSecrets website.

children's health, and the planet's health. It would be ideal to be able to rely on the government's help...but, as you've already noticed, unfortunately, the government has too many of its interests tied up with mega-corporations, which is why the change has to start with us: with consumer strength.

If you feel it's time to make a transformation, the first step is to modify the way you relate to what you eat and replicate these changes within your family, your friends, and your community. To make this change happen, we need to recognize that our consumption habits are rooted to the need for instant gratification. By becoming aware of this need, we create space for acting mindfully and recognizing the consequences of our actions in the future. If we take advantage of our true consumer power, we can make the impact of these changes go viral through social media. It's been witnessed repeatedly that when social movements like this are sparked, corporations have no other choice but to reinvent themselves and start doing the right thing...otherwise...they'll meet their end...

We still have time to turn the environmental and health crisis around. If we recognize the importance of our role as consumers, not only will we have an impact at home, but we can also unleash a true social change that will attract the attention of governments and corporations. For example, if you make a small change at home that represents 1% of your habitual practices, and then your family and friends replicate it and also promote it among their groups and communities, and then finally an entire population adopts it, then the total accumulated change will be tremendous.

Remember the 9 billion animals that are killed for consumption each year in the United States? If the country were to reduce its consumption of animal products by just 1%, we could save up to 90 million animals a year—not a negligible sum—that, undoubtedly, would contribute to reducing the environmental impact of industrial farms. According to the World Economic Forum report from February 2019,[47] globally, 50 billion poultry, 1.5 billion pigs, and 500 million sheep are killed for human consumption each year. Likewise, according to various reviews from Faunalytics dated October 2018, the figures for cows and goats are 300 million and 450 million, respectively. Based on these studies, of the countries that killed the highest number of livestock in 2016, China was first in line, with nearly 50 million, followed by Brazil, the U.S., Argentina, and India.[48] Worldwide, each year we kill around 53 billion animals for human consumption (that's right, fifty-three billion animals and this figure does not include marine animals). If we were to make a tiny change in our diets by reducing that figure by 1%, we could save 530 million land animals. This 1%, which seems like a trivial number in our lives, would considerably reduce our environmental footprint and, while it's an insignificant change for each of us individually, the overall accumulated result is extraordinary.

Consumer strength is immense. We just have to take the first step and decide to make a small change that can be replicated. We've run out of the time and justifications needed to sit back with our arms crossed waiting for someone else to get an idea that might return the future we have stolen…

---

[47] https://www.weforum.org/agenda/2019/02/chart-of-the-day-this-is-how-many-animals-we-eat-each-year/
[48] https://faunalytics.org/global-cow-slaughter-statistics-and-charts/

❧ 6 ❧

FEAR OF CHANGE

HE WHO IS WITHOUT SIN MAY CAST THE FIRST STONE...

I have a confession to make…

Even though I've transitioned toward a WFPB diet (remember, this isn't a swear word, but rather the initials for Whole Food Plant-Based), I'm still not 100% there, and I must confess that I have a guilty pleasure: cheese. That's right, every now and then, I eat cheese. And the thing is, the goal of changing your eating habits is not about becoming the Mother Teresa of nutrition. We have to start by making easier changes that will start to clear our paths so we can face the ones that are harder for us. The way I took on this change was by eliminating all products of animal origin from my diet, except cheese. However, I have a few rules that are part of my policy: The cheese should be made in Europe (because the use of rBGH has been banned there), and I can only eat it once a day and, at most, three or four times a week. This is what I've chosen as my personal policy, and it's what has worked for me in this transition process.

YOUR PERSONAL POLICY

It doesn't really matter who you believe you are, how you define yourself, or how others define you: the truth is that you are constantly changing because, ideally, you are always trying to find balance. Yet, balance is not a static point—it's dynamic, as dynamic as life itself. Imagine a tightrope walker, an acrobat balancing on a wire. Or how about we take it even further: Imagine Philippe Petit that cold morning of August 7, 1974, when he crossed the distance between the rooftops of the World Trade Center's Twin Towers in New York walking on a cable at 1,362 feet (415 meters) above ground. He didn't just cross one time but eight, while he danced, laughed, and did tricks on the tightrope to the amazement and disbelief of his spectators. He had such great control over his body that he watched a seagull as it flew around his head and even poked fun at the NYPD officers who were there waiting for him to finish so they could arrest him after his last walk across to the south tower.[49] Now, imagine that the tightrope is life and you are Philippe. Of course, while walking along the tightrope, it would be necessary to analyze your positioning second by second along with the way you're leaning and your weight in order to constantly rebalance and compensate. If you're shifted to the left, you would immediately have to correct to the right, but not too much—or too little—since you could lose your balance again. Analyzing, compensating, and readjusting would become an endless task, an automatic activity…otherwise, you would fall. What I'm saying is: balance is not static. It demands constant analysis, evaluation, and adjustment. To get in the flow and find harmony, our lifestyle should be based on this

---

[49] You can see a Ted Talk about his experiences as a magician and high-wire artist here: https://www.youtube.com/watch?v=k3zZVQPaKKQ&list=TLPQMDkwNDIwMjAPUdI YJuhrZQ&index=2

same dynamism, in endless motion. Yet, I've heard arguments stating that the healthy thing to do is to find the middle ground, which only leaves the question: "A middle ground of what?"

Where is the middle ground when we feel like individuals who are separate from the rest of the world and whose only concern is to attend to our personal needs? And, in contrast, where is the middle ground when we feel like we are part of something larger than ourselves and we're aiming for the common good? The term *middle ground* is deceiving because it depends on our circumstances, our observations, and our personal story. It also depends on the way we interpret the world, which is absolutely subjective. When we persistently defend that it's ideal to find middle ground in our diets, what we actually mean is that we are not willing to change our way of life. To the contrary, if we stop to think and analyze the best way to find balance, we'll reach the conclusion that if we just stand still on the tightrope, we'll end up losing balance and falling into the abyss. That's right, we need constant balance, motion, and adaptation, and then it will dawn on us that it's not about middle ground—it's about living in the present and observing the precise moment to understand where we need to distribute our weight to and how we should direct our strength in order to take the next step. In the early 20th century, solving the health problems of the world's population entailed promoting and providing animal protein to all social strata. That action was necessary to keep things in balance during that period. But today, life is completely different. The world population, food production mechanisms, health services, and technology are not like they were a century ago. It's time to analyze where we are and what's happening around us, and then make the necessary changes to, once again, find harmony with the world we live in.

Change is an opportunity to grow and face our deepest fears, and we have all experienced it to a greater or lesser extent. We experience it when we get hired to our first job; we yearn for it when we decide to live our life with a partner; it turns our life upside down when our first baby is born; it shows us our hidden strength if we have to move to another country; it fills us with joy if our quality of life improves; and it devastates us when we lose a loved one. Change is a constant in anyone's life, and, if we learn to appreciate it, it reveals the magnitude of our inner strength and what we are capable of. Change is also incredibly useful to us when we need to adapt to uncertainty through mental flexibility, creativity, and resilience. There are some changes that we decide to make on our own, and others come to us as part of the process of life. When we decide to make a change, the journey should be more important than the destination. The idea is to make small adjustments that translate into big transformations. In this process, we should not focus on reaching perfection, but rather on improving what can be improved and is within our possibilities. In most cases, it is beneficial to steer clear of radicalizing our opinions.

If we decide to make changes to our eating habits, avoiding extremes is a good idea. We shouldn't think of our diets as being something totally perfect (for example: 100% free of animal products) or something totally imperfect (for example: 100% animal products)– or vice versa. Between these two extremes, there is a wide spectrum of levels: pick the level that makes you feel better and, from there, keep moving toward the end of the spectrum that is free of animal products. It's not about eliminating these products all at once or once and for all. It's about changing portion sizes, including more (unprocessed) fruits and vegetables, and returning to our local and traditional diets, which are in tune with the planet's resources. You can invent your own personal policy, too. Test what works for you and what doesn't. This may mean leaving behind dairy products (especially if you want to lose weight). Another option is to set apart one day each week when you don't eat animal products. Or in your case it might be switching from eating bacon and eggs for breakfast to having a fruit and vegetable smoothy or perhaps substituting the meat in your dishes with mushrooms or lentils. I know someone who organized his personal policy like this: zero animal products in the morning and part of the afternoon, but after 6:00 p.m., he can have whatever he feels like eating. Other people have switched up the order of their dishes, starting with a large salad that makes them feel almost completely satisfied from the beginning of the meal.

It's important for you to keep making changes that get you closer to the other end of the spectrum, perhaps with a small step each month or perhaps with a little bigger jump every year. If you achieve a small 5% change this year, added to another small change the next, the transformation for your life, for the planet, and for future generations will be significant. Imagine what a 5% change in the entire population would do for the environment on a global level! But the change is yours to make—it's in your hands. Define your personal policy in a way that works well for you and make your best effort to fulfill it. If necessary, seek out help from nutrition specialists (doctors, nutritionists, or integrative health coaches) who share your same concerns for the planet's future, your health, and the health of your loved ones. Be sure to let the change be self-driven, though, —rather than imposed—to allow for the transformation to soak into your conscience and your children's conscience. Do what's best for you, but start by doing something right now.

If at some point you can't comply with your personal policy, it's okay—it's not a diet written in stone, you're not a bad person, you're not throwing away all your previous efforts. Don't label yourself. It doesn't mean that your policy is bad or that you're not taking interest in it. Keep a positive focus on continuing to make your way through the spectrum. Some experts say that in 50 to 100 years all human beings will have a plant-based diet. Whether this happens as the result of a catastrophe or due to a peaceful transformation that favors life will depend on 1) us making the right decisions today and 2) our commitment as a society to make a change that the planet urgently needs.

LET'S DREAM BIG

In no way would I dare deny that products of animal origin provide human beings with certain nutrients and played an essential role in the health of humanity in the early 20th century. Today, while it's true that we can benefit from their nutritional qualities, the problem is that the amount of animal products we consume by far exceeds the recommended portions. According to a study conducted by the United States Department of Agriculture (USDA) based on statistics from 2017,[50] the average American's consumption of meat, eggs, and dairy products exceeded the recommendations established in the nutritional guidelines by 40% (the maximum is 155 grams of products of animal origin a day for an adult).[51] Since the 1960s, the average weight for humans has increased by 20% (in the 1960s, the average weight had already significantly increased in comparison to the average weight in the early 20th century). It's true that people today are bigger, but it's hard not to wonder the same thing Michael Pollan has questioned about whether this means people are healthier.

When added to the low-quality nutrients in products from animals raised on industrial farms and the toxic load that they have bioaccumulated, it's just not worth the damage we are doing to the planet, the deterioration of our health, the increased inequality, the mistreatment of other living beings, or the obvious theft of resources from future generations. The food industry—which protects itself by hiding under arguments of the generous work it does to offer humanity large quantities of macronutrients to satiate hunger—has manipulated

---

[50] https://www.ers.usda.gov/data-products/ag-and-food-statistics-charting-the-essentials/food-availability-and-consumption/
[51] https://www.dietaryguidelines.gov/sites/default/files/2019-05/2015-2020_Dietary_Guidelines.pdf

our consumption patterns in such a way over the past century that our ingestion of cheap animal origin products, subsidized by the government, has become excessive. The fact of the matter is that the way we eat today is very different from the way human beings ate up until relatively recently, and this change in our customs and behaviors is strongly linked to what the government subsidizes...or...doesn't subsidize...

Optimal health goes beyond a lack of illness because it implies total well-being in all spheres of life: physical, mental, emotional, social, and spiritual. Sadly, our modern health-care system is specifically based on treating the symptoms of diseases but not on preventing them, and much less on analyzing the conditions that cause them. Our modern times have us tethered in a vicious circle in which we eat products that make us sick and then seek out medical care to get a miraculous pill or treatment that quickly hides the symptoms. Meanwhile, we ignore its actual causes. And in truth, as long as we keep consuming products that make us sick and ignoring the biological and environmental factors that contribute to our current illnesses, we will continue to live half-heartedly, sick, and with low quality of life. It's worth remembering that taxpayers are the ones who cover public health expenses. Our taxes pay for everything from lung damage caused by smoking to the costs of addressing obesity and diabetes—a result of a society addicted to fats and sugars—to the cardiovascular damage brought on by abusing food of animal origin. Today, the individualist thinking of "I'll do whatever I want with my health" is no longer valid. Our right to harm ourselves ends when someone else (society, the government, our children, or our grandchildren) has to cover the costs.

We can't keep waiting for governments or corporations to solve the extremely serious problems in public health and environmental deterioration: no amount of money will be enough to solve these problems if, as a society, we don't attack them at their roots. We should start with what we put on our plates and our children's plates. And the dilemma doesn't lie so much in the food we do eat but rather in the food we've stopped eating, provided that—with guidance from nutrition experts whose approach is solely focused on nutrients—the presence of unprocessed fruits and vegetables in meals is currently next to none. (They're often considered a garnish.) Copying the convenient—but unsustainable and unhealthy—Standard American Diet (SAD) has made us dismiss the nutritional value that foods of plant origin can provide in our meals. The global effect has been a trend of ignoring and pushing aside traditional and local diets. Three in every four American children leave out their daily helpings of fruits and vegetables and eat more saturated fats than the portions recommended in dietary guidelines.

From a place of heightened awareness, perhaps it's worth asking yourself: *"What are my children eating?"* Depending on the answer, consider if the time has come to put aside beliefs that your family, friends, doctors, the mass media, and even the government have been repeating. Go back in time. If your grandparents are still alive and well, ask them what their diets consisted of when they were kids. Do some research and form your own conclusions. The mass media has been conditioning us for many years, and it's time to start asking ourselves what it is that really makes us feel well, to analyze our behavior, and to decide what path we will take. Isn't it strange that despite the incredible technological advancements in the field of medicine, a large part of the world population lives in a state of chronic illness? Our current situation is the result of an unfortunate combination of factors: 1) the degradation and contamination of our natural resources, 2) an excessive increase in the consumption of animal products, 3) the low consumption of products of plant origin, and 4) the radical change in our lifestyles. If you want to make a change that will transform your life, the lives of your loved ones, and the lives of future generations in a positive way, my recommendation is to start by listening to yourself. By reading your own body, try to sense what's right and what makes you feel well. What I'm proposing is not a campaign against consuming products of animal origin. My proposal is just to put more servings of fruits and vegetables on our plates, reduce the huge quantity of animal products that we consume every day, and improve the quality of the nutrients in those foods.

One of the last projects I reviewed when I was working at the environmental fund was focused on the environmental benefits that regenerative ranching offers. The overall idea is to allow livestock to graze freely in paddocks that are periodically rotated in order to use some pasture areas while others are allowed to rest for up to a year. In certain ecosystems and climates, such as the grasslands of northern Mexico, this rotation helps soil to naturally regenerate and does not require fertilizers or chemical products during the restoration cycle. This ranching model brings about significant environmental benefits: 1) The livestock grazes—that is, it eats its natural food and is not given any kind of antibiotic. Accordingly, its excrement transforms into an important part of the cycle of sustainable regeneration (contrary to the excrement on industrial farms that turns into a contaminant), involving everything from microorganisms and insects (such as beetles, which play a crucial role) to birds and mammals. This is an excellent model of environmental circularity in which there is no waste, but rather everything becomes critical raw material for the process. 2) The livestock can walk around freely and, by doing so, they work the ground, aerating it and making it permeable, allowing the aquifers to replenish and preventing the soil from turning into a hard, cracked and dry layer, which is what we see when it erodes. 3) The livestock, as an active part of the cycle, is healthy and needs fewer vaccines (in some cases, none). Regenerative practices, as opposed to the standard practices that we see on industrial farms, respect the soil, water, air, biological diversity, and natural cycles of ecosystems. Regenerative livestock contributes to absorbing the carbon that is present in the atmosphere in order to integrate it into the soil, commonly known as carbon capturing, which makes it possible to reverse the effects of climate change. This results in breeding healthy and strong animals that are treated with dignity and whose products offer humans more and better nutritional content.

We should also return to traditional agricultural practices, those that have a deep respect for the Earth and recognize the importance of the interdependence of different species. Small-scale sustainable practices (which depend on people and not machines and are based on biological farming methods, not chemical ones) increase soil fertility and health, which increases its capacity to store or capture carbon. If carbon is stored in soil, then it can't be released into the atmosphere. Unfortunately, mono and dual crops are just as damaging and unsustainable as industrial farms. If we don't change this form of agriculture, it's been predicted that it will be the source of pests that will be very difficult to fight off in a not-so-distant future. The way we behave as a social group is the force that will obligate the industry to refocus agriculture into farming diverse species that provide human beings with high nutritional value.

After four years of study and research, the International Assessment of Agricultural Science and Technology for Development (IAASTD), whose final report was signed by the governments of 57 countries, established that the only solution for offsetting the counterproductive effects of our agricultural production model is to channel our efforts toward establishing agroecological systems that reduce the use of agrochemicals and fossil fuels (synthetic fertilizers and pesticides). The only way to meet this goal is by respecting the biological diversity of ecosystems.

Our responsibility as consumers is to ensure that our consumable goods come from small-scale farms and ranches that foster the sustainable management of resources, environmental circularity, and carbon capturing. Let's take advantage of the power behind our decision to demand that the products we buy be quality products. Let's promote the consumption of foods that come from regenerative or holistic farms that, in addition to offering benefits of protecting and caring for the environment, activate the economies of many rural communities. If we make this small change, the results will have a ripple effect and cause a positive impact on different fronts. It will:

✓ Moderate the consumption of quality products of animal origin.

✓ Foster agriculture and ranching practices based on regenerative models and environmental circularity that play a critical role in reversing the effects of climate change (through carbon capturing).

✓ Reduce the use of synthetic, fossil-fuel based fertilizers and pesticides through practices focused on recovering ecosystems' biological diversity.

✓ End intensive agricultural practices and those involving the chemical or genetic modification of cereals, grains, legumes, and seeds.

✓ Restore and regenerate degraded ecosystems.

What could be a better gift for our children?

❧ 7 ❧

NOW WHAT DO I DO?

WHO AM I?

Many people have asked me: When you go to a restaurant, why do you say you're vegan instead of vegetarian? (Remember that I still eat some cheese.) I tell them that, honestly, I don't consider myself to be either one, but it's much easier to explain to a waiter that I'm vegan but it's okay if the dish has a little cheese or honey than to say I'm vegetarian, but my dish shouldn't include eggs, or milk, or cream, or yogurt. Ultimately, they're nothing more than labels—they help us understand how the world works and our relationship with it, but they don't define us.

And I'm going to tell you the same thing: don't let labels define you. Make the changes that make you feel well. When you change something in your lifestyle, it's common for people to poke fun and question your intentions, but keep in mind that it's not about getting wrapped up in the glamor or let-downs of the latest trends, which, once again, are nothing more than labels. It's about starting to act from the heart. It's quite hard to define who we are because we think our personal backgrounds and the labels we've put on ourselves are who we are. Don't worry, I won't start philosophizing, but what

I can tell you is that you are a beautiful, unique, and unrepeatable being who came into this world to fulfill a purpose. What is it? Only you can know. Some ancient texts say that arriving in this world as a human being is one of the greatest privileges of creation, so it's not so ridiculous to think that you can fulfill this unique and special purpose while leaving a trail of light in your wake. In most cases, big changes start with small actions. A small act of kindness can lead to an extraordinary transformation in the person (or being) who receives it, who can, in turn, replicate it. This first action has the potential to be repeated perpetually (like a rock tossed in the water that creates ripples on the surface). So, never waste an opportunity to shine.

In some cultures, the same word is used for both "problem" and "opportunity." In reality, life is neutral. What happens is neither good nor bad. Life doesn't happen to you, it just happens. You have the power to view any situation as a problem or an opportunity. What's marvelous is that you (and you alone) have the authority to make the decision and adjust to the conditions that present themselves to you. You can view the environmental and health crisis as a problem you can't do anything about because you feel small and insignificant, or you can see it as an opportunity to try out your creativity, resilience, and mental flexibility.

If you decide to view these challenges as opportunities for transformation—instead of having a presence in the world of "just passing through" —you will leave a profound mark by making the changes that future generations need.

DELICIOUS RECIPES FOR A SIMPLE TRANSITION

Perhaps you're thinking: "I agree. You've convinced me, and I understand that, by reducing my consumption of animal products, I can do my small part in the effort to reverse environmental deterioration. But now, what are we going to eat at my house?" The same thing happened to me. Suddenly, I was lost in the kitchen between ingredients that tasted like cardboard and absolute confusion.

Maybe you've reduced your use of plastics. You might have invested in solar panels or in a hybrid vehicle. Perhaps you've changed out your traditional lightbulbs for ones that are energy efficient, and of course you separate your trash. How about eating a salad instead of a hamburger?

There's something we shouldn't forget here: Eating is pleasurable. Meals should be a pleasant moment for sharing time with others, for showing self-love, for getting in touch with the fruits of nature and, certainly, for bringing delight to our eyes and tastebuds. Some time ago, a friend told me he believed that the most efficient way to feed humanity—to avoid doing more damage to the planet while also fighting all forms of malnutrition (which includes both undernutrition and overnutrition)—would be to put our food into smoothies and bars with high nutritional content. But this would mean that the joy of eating and sharing time together at meals would be lost. Moreover, as we've discussed throughout the book, nothing can substitute the nutrients that come in their original packaging: real food.

I don't think it's necessary to reach these extremes if we start making conscious changes to our food choices. As I've been saying all throughout this book, it's not about stuffing our bodies with isolated nutrients. For example, it's known that antioxidants work when we eat them in their original packaging (fruits and vegetables), but there are also studies which conclude that, when isolated, these same antioxidants can cause cancer. Why insist on manipulating nutrients to isolate them when the Earth has already integrated them into the foods it provides for us and that, in their natural forms, are also the best allies for our health? I can't think of any better food than the food that was designed over the course of thousands of years and has been there in our evolutionary process to provide us with the specific nutrients that our bodies and our microbiomes need.

The magic of food is in its vivid colors that invite us to taste it, in its texture and consistency that make us close our eyes in pleasure, and in its delicious smells that makes our mouths water. The purpose of food is to satisfy our hunger, but also our spirits. We should touch it, feel it, and smell it so that, when we take the first bite, it makes us vibrate… And that's how we can truly define it as food: because it excites us, because we enjoy it, and it makes us feel happy.

And best of all, it's there for us because the Earth gives it to us. Her fruits grow and ripen for us. Let's turn to see the true food, the food that has life, the food that gets its nutrients from fertile soil and grows with the sun's energy, the food that doesn't need packaging or promoting, and that shares information with our cells and microbiomes.

Let's return to our roots, to what we really are, to the essence of our humanity: to being one with Mother Earth…

Let's eat!

On the pages that follow, you'll find 16 delicious vegan recipes that chef Natalia Delgado prepared exclusively for this book. Natalia is a self-proclaimed environmental activist, and her wish is to teach the world to adopt a lifestyle that's in harmony with the planet through her splendid vegan cuisine. As an internationally renowned chef, author, and expert, she has been invited repeatedly to speak at culinary festivals around the world. What's more, she has also been the host and producer of a variety of cooking programs.

When you prepare these recipes, not only will you be doing your small part to make the world a better place, but you'll also be surprised by how delicious meals from a diet free of animal products can be. To add to this, chef Natalia's recipes are a feast of colors, flavors, textures, and seasoning that will leave your family wanting more.

You can find even more delicious recipes on her Facebook page and Instagram account.

A note about the recipes:

As I said at the beginning of the book, there are foods that are ideal for some people but harmful to others. The recipes presented here are meant to make you feel well and happy. Don't hesitate to change any of the ingredients. For example, if you have a peanut allergy, you can use other nuts like almonds, pine nuts, macadamia nuts, pecans, walnuts, or cashews. Some people don't digest cucumber well, in which case you can substitute it with a summer squash like zucchini. If chickpeas aren't your thing, in the hummus recipe, you can replace them with haricot or pinto beans. As a health coach, I suggest that when a recipe says "vegetable oil" you use coconut oil because it contains lauric acid, which has antipathogenic properties. The final choice is up to you, though, depending on what makes you feel well.

Lastly, the idea is for you to have fun, to enjoy the colors, flavors, and textures of the dishes, but, above all, for them to contribute to your "well-being." Explore your kitchen and your tastes. Start to recognize and get to know which foods work well for you.

Bon appetit!

HUMMUS WITH SERRANO CHILI PEPPER

Ingredients:

1 serrano chili pepper
2 cups cooked chickpeas
2 cloves of garlic
3 Tbsp. lemon juice
2 Tbsp. tahini (sesame paste)
  or sesame oil
3 Tbsp. olive oil
1 tsp. cumin
1 tsp. salt
1 small handful of sesame
  seeds

Steps:

1. Heat a griddle and roast
   the chili pepper until it's
   soft and browned; take
   out the seeds.
2. Combine the ingredients
   in a food processor until
   they become a soft paste.
3. Garnish with toasted
   sesame seeds and a splash
   of olive oil.
4. Serve with pita bread and
   your choice of vegetables.

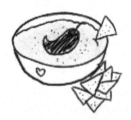

Spring Rolls with Mango and Avocado

Ingredients.

12 sheets of rice paper
1 cup baby spinach
1 avocado, thinly sliced
1 mango, thinly sliced
Fresh cilantro
1 cup grated carrots
½ cup grated purple cabbage
2 spring onions, cut into
  strips

For the peanut sauce:

½ cup peanut butter
3 Tbsp. rice vinegar
2 Tbsp. tamari sauce (gluten
  free soy sauce)
1 garlic clove, grated
1 Tbsp. Thai-style hot sauce
  (Sriracha)
1 tsp. ginger powder

Steps.

1. Mix the sauce ingredients in a bowl, combining them well. Set aside.
2. Heat ½ cup of water and pour it onto a long plate.

   Note: The water should be lukewarm (not too hot) because the sheets of rice paper can get too soft. The rice paper will remain moist from the residual heat on the cutting board.

3. Quickly, dip a sheet of rice paper in the water and then place it on a cutting board. Pile a handful of spinach leaves on top of the rice paper, adding a little avocado, several slices of mango, cilantro leaves, carrot, purple cabbage, and onion.
4. Fold in the edges and shape into a roll. Cut in half and serve with sauce.

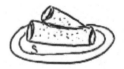

POTATO TOMATO SOUP

Ingredients:	Steps:
3 Tbsp. olive oil 3 peeled potatoes (russet) cut into strips ½ tsp. salt Pepper to taste 2 ripe tomatoes, grated (1 cup) ½ onion, grated 3 cups vegetable broth 1 green California (Anaheim) chili, chopped into slices	1. Heat a pot on high and add the oil and potatoes. Sauté for 1 minute, stirring constantly so they don't brown. 2. Add salt and pepper. Sauté for 30 seconds longer. 3. Add the tomato and onion and cook for 1 minute. 4. Add the vegetable broth and chili pepper. Cover and cook over medium heat for 8 minutes until the potato is soft. 5. Serve warm.

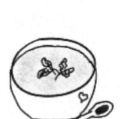

JICAMA AND MANGO CEVICHE

Ingredients:

2 mangos, ripe but still firm,
  cut into cubes
2 cups jicama, cut into cubes
1 cucumber cut into cubes
  without seeds
1 red bell pepper, chopped
½ red onion, chopped
1 serrano chili pepper,
  chopped
2 carrots, grated
¼ cup cilantro, chopped
½ cup lime juice
3 Tbsp. tamari sauce
1 Tbsp. tabasco sauce
3 Tbsp. olive oil
1 tsp. salt

To serve:
Avocado, cut into cubes

Steps:

1. Mix the ingredients in a bowl
    and refrigerate until the
    mixture is well chilled.

Note. It is very important to
serve this dish cold. Temperature
plays a key role in our food.

2. Before serving, add an
    avocado cut into cubes.
3. Serve and enjoy.

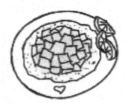

BROWN RICE WITH PINEAPPLE AND PEANUTS

Ingredients:

4 cups cooked brown rice
2 Tbsp. sesame oil
½ red onion, chopped
1 garlic clove, minced
1 Tbsp. fresh, grated ginger
1 cup chopped broccoli
1 cup chopped baby corn
1 bell pepper, chopped
1 cup chopped pineapple
2 spring onions, chopped
¼ cup chopped cilantro
1 cup toasted peanuts
4 Tbsp. tamari sauce
2 Tbsp. lime juice
1 tsp. salt

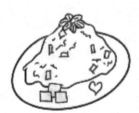

Steps:

To cook the rice:

1. Put 2 cups of brown rice in a wire strainer and rinse it with water.
2. Add the rice to a pot with 4½ cups of water. Bring to a boil and cover. Reduce to low heat and cook for 20 minutes.
3. Turn off the heat and uncover. Stir with a fork.
4. Cover again and let sit for 10 minutes.

For the dish:

1. Heat a wok or a large saucepan. Add the oil, onion, garlic, and ginger and cook for several seconds.
2. Add the broccoli, baby corn, bell pepper, pineapple, spring onions, cilantro, and peanuts. Stir, cooking for 2 minutes.
3. Add the rice, tamari sauce, lime juice, and salt. Mix and cook for 2 minutes.
4. Add the cilantro, spring onion, and peanuts.
5. Serve and enjoy.

CREAM OF BROCCOLI SOUP WITH SUNFLOWER SEEDS

Ingredients:

3 cups broccoli
½ white or yellow onion
4 cups vegetable broth, divided
1 cup sunflower seeds
2 Tbsp. olive oil
1 Tbsp. corn or potato starch
1 tsp. salt
½ tsp. black pepper

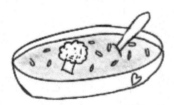

Steps:

1. Add the broccoli and onion to a pot with 3 cups of the vegetable broth. Cover and cook over medium heat for 15 minutes.
2. Set aside ¼ cup of cooked broccoli and mince it.
3. Combine the remaining broccoli with the cooked onion in the blender. Add the sunflower seeds along with the cup of broth that you had set aside. Blend for 4 minutes until the mixture is soft and creamy and place it in a heated pot with the olive oil.
4. Dissolve the corn or potato starch in two tablespoons of cold water and add it to the soup.
5. Add the salt and pepper, then let it thicken for 5 minutes.
6. Add the minced broccoli that you had set aside.
7. Serve and enjoy.

LENTIL PICADILLO

Ingredients:

2 Tbsp. olive oil
½ onion, chopped
1 garlic clove, minced
2 carrots, chopped
2 potatoes, cut into cubes
2 ripe tomatoes, chopped
1 cup tomato puree or ripe,
   grated tomato
1 cup vegetable broth
2 cups cooked lentils (al
   dente)
1 tsp. oregano
2 Tbsp. cilantro, chopped
1 tsp. salt
¾ cup green olives, sliced
2 Tbsp. apple vinegar

To serve:

Avocado
Limes

Steps:

1. Heat the oil and sauté the onion and garlic, then add the carrots, potatoes, and tomato. Cook for 3 minutes.
2. Add the puree, broth, cooked lentils (*al dente*), oregano, cilantro, and salt. Cover over low heat for 10 minutes until the potatoes are cooked.

NOTE: *Al dente* means that it is not over cooked (because it will turn into a puree) or under cooked (because they'll be hard). This is a term that's used for pasta and legumes.

3. Uncover and add the olives and vinegar. Cook for 3 minutes.
4. Serve with avocado and limes.

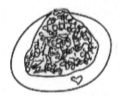

OYSTER MUSHROOM TACOS AL PASTOR WITH SALSA VERDE

Ingredients:

2 Tbsp. olive oil
½ onion, sliced in wedges
3 cups of oyster mushrooms, shredded
½ tsp. salt

For the marinade:

1 guajillo chili pepper, rehydrated
¼ onion, cooked
1 garlic clove
½ cup vegetable broth
1 Tbsp. achiote paste
1 tsp. cumin
1 tsp. oregano
2 Tbsp. apple vinegar
½ cup orange juice

To serve:

Tortillas
Lettuce leaves
Roasted pineapple
Chopped onion
Chopped cilantro

Salsa verde:

10 tomatillos, cooked
3 serrano chili peppers, cooked
¼ cup cilantro
1 garlic clove
1 Tbsp. apple vinegar
1 Tbsp. salt

Steps:

1. Blend the ingredients for the marinade together and set aside.
2. Add the oil and onions to a skillet and cook for 1 minute over high heat. Add the shredded oyster mushrooms and cook for 2 minutes, then add the salt, toasting them slightly.
3. Add the marinade and cook for 5 minutes until the sauce reduces and thickens.
4. Serve as tacos in tortillas or lettuce leaves with roasted pineapple, onion, cilantro, and salsa verde.

Note: To rehydrate the guajillo chili pepper, place it in hot water and wait 10 minutes.

Salsa verde:

Put the ingredients in a blender and blend for 1 minute.

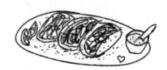

SAUTÉED BROCCOLI WITH CASHEWS

Ingredients:

2 Tbsp. olive oil
½ onion, chopped
1 cup broccoli
1 cup sliced mushrooms
2 sticks of celery, chopped
1 bell pepper, cut in strips
1 zucchini squash, chopped
1 garlic clove, minced
2 Tbsp. tamari sauce
1 cup cashews (unchopped)
1 Tbsp. black sesame seeds

TO SERVE:
Brown jasmine rice, steamed

Steps:

1. Add the oil, onion, and vegetables to a very hot skillet.
2. Stir quickly, sautéing for several seconds.
3. Add the garlic and sauté constantly for 2 minutes.
4. Add the tamari sauce and, cashews and cook for 3 minutes.
5. It's ready! Serve over steamed rice and sprinkle with black sesame seeds.

NOTE: The vegetables should be crunchy and brightly colored. You can use whatever vegetables you have available.

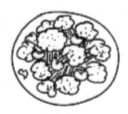

CURRIED LENTILS WITH SPINACH

Ingredients:

1½ cups lentils
4 cups vegetable broth
1 garlic clove, minced
1 bay leaf
1 cup tomato puree or ripe grated tomato
3 Tbsp. grated onion (white or yellow)
1 Tbsp. curry powder
1 tsp. salt
1 cup Thai-style coconut milk
2 cups chopped spinach
3 Tbsp. chopped cilantro

Steps:

1. Add the lentils to a pot with the broth, garlic, and bay leaf. Cover and cook over low heat for 20 minutes.
2. Add the tomato puree, onion, curry powder, and salt. Cook for 5 minutes.
3. Add the coconut milk, spinach, and cilantro. Cook for 3 minutes.
4. Serve and enjoy.

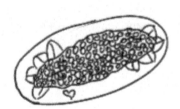

TANDOORI CAULIFLOWER

Ingredients:

¼ cup olive oil
3 Tbsp. lime juice
1 tsp. curry powder
½ cup Thai-style coconut milk
1 garlic clove, grated
1 tsp. paprika powder
1 head of cauliflower

For the sauce:

1 Tbsp. olive oil
1 garlic clove, grated
1 Tbsp. fresh, grated ginger
1 tsp. curry powder
1 cup Thai-style coconut milk
2 Tbsp. cilantro, chopped
1 tsp. salt

Serve with:

Chopped cilantro
Almonds, sliced or chopped

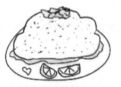

Steps:

1. Preheat the oven to 375°F/175°C.
2. Mix the olive oil, lime juice, curry, coconut milk, garlic, and paprika together in a bowl.
3. Place the head of cauliflower on a baking pan and spread the mixture over the cauliflower.
4. Put the cauliflower in the oven for 25 minutes until it browns.
5. Cut the cauliflower and serve it with cilantro and almonds.

For the sauce:

1. Heat a pot over medium heat, then add the oil and sauté the garlic and ginger for 30 seconds. Add the curry powder and cook for 30 seconds longer.
2. Add the coconut milk and cook for 5 minutes over low heat. Add the cilantro and salt and cook for 30 seconds.
3. Serve with the roasted cauliflower.

FALAFEL WITH CREAMY AVOCADO SAUCE

Ingredients:	Steps:
2 cups chickpeas, soaked for 8 hours (not cooked)	1. Soak chickpeas overnight (8 hours) in a bowl with 4 cups of water.
¼ cup parsley	
¼ cup cilantro	2. Drain the water off the chickpeas and add them to the remaining ingredients in a food processor or blender, mixing them until they form a paste.
1 garlic clove	
¼ onion	
1 Tbsp. salt	
1 tsp. baking soda	
1 tsp. cumin	
2 Tbsp. lime juice	3. Shape the falafel into 2½ inch (6 cm) balls.
4 Tbsp. crushed oats (can be substituted with chickpea flour)	4. Heat the oil over medium-high heat, then dip the falafel balls in it, frying them for 3 to 4 minutes until they brown.
½ cup frying oil	

For the avocado sauce:

1 ripe avocado
1 tsp. tamari sauce
2 Tbsp. cilantro
3 Tbsp. lime juice
1 garlic clove
1 serrano chili pepper
2 Tbsp. sesame oil
1 pinch of cumin

5. Take them out and let them drip for several seconds. Serve immediately afterward with the salsa.

Note: Instead of frying, they can also be baked at 395°F/200°C for 25 minutes.

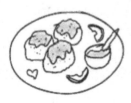

For the avocado sauce:

Add the ingredients to the blender, processing until they form a creamy sauce. Serve with the falafel.

LETTUCE TACOS WITH PEANUT SAUCE

Ingredients:

2 Tbsp. sesame oil
½ onion, chopped
1 garlic glove, minced
1 Tbsp. grated ginger
3 cups chopped button
  mushrooms
1 cup chopped peanuts
1 Tbsp. corn or potato starch
¼ cup vegetable broth
1 Tbsp. rice vinegar
¼ cup cilantro
4 spring onions, chopped
3 Tbsp. tamari sauce

For the peanut sauce:

½ cup toasted peanuts
2 Tbsp. tamari sauce
¼ cup rice vinegar
1 garlic clove
2 Tbsp. Thai-style hot sauce
  (Sriracha)
½ cup water

To serve:

Lettuce leaves
Chopped purple cabbage
Cilantro
Peanuts

Steps:

1. Add the oil, onion, garlic, and ginger to a heated saucepan and sauté for 30 seconds. Add the mushrooms and peanuts and cook for 3 minutes.

2. Dissolve the starch in the broth and vinegar and then add it to the saucepan along with the cilantro, spring onion, and tamari sauce. Allow it to thicken.

3. Put the ingredients for the peanut sauce in the blender. Blend and serve in a bowl.

4. Make tacos with the lettuce leaves, add the sauce and garnishes.

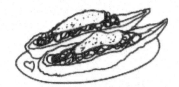

OYSTER MUSHROOM SALAD

Ingredients:

3 Tbsp. olive oil
4 cups shredded oyster
mushrooms
1 garlic clove, minced
2 Tbsp. tamari sauce
1 tsp. salt

For the salad:

1 red onion, sliced in wedges
4 tomatillos, chopped
without seeds
2 serrano chili peppers,
chopped
1 cup chopped olives
1 cup chopped radishes
1 cup cilantro leaves
2 avocados, cut into cubes
3 cups chopped lettuce

For the vinaigrette:

¼ cup vegetable broth
¼ cup lime juice
¼ cup olive oil
1 tsp. oregano
1 Tbsp. salt
2 Tbsp. red wine vinegar

Steps:

1. Add oil and oyster
   mushrooms to a hot skillet
   and cook for 3 minutes.
2. Add the garlic and the
   tamari sauce. Cook for 5
   minutes.
3. Add the salt and cook for 2
   minutes until browned.
4. Let them cool completely.

For the vinaigrette:

In a small bowl, mix all the
ingredients for the vinaigrette.

For the salad:

In a bowl, mix the oyster
mushrooms with all the
remaining ingredients except
for the lettuce.
Add the vinaigrette and
refrigerate for 1 hour.
Add the lettuce, mix, and
serve.

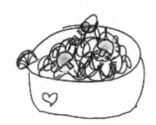

OATMEAL BANANA MUFFINS WITH CHOCOLATE CHIPS

Ingredients:

2 tsp. baking powder
1 tsp. baking soda
2 cups crushed oats
2 ripe bananas, mashed
1 tsp. vanilla
½ cup agave nectar or pure maple syrup
1 cup unsweetened plant-based milk
3 Tbsp. peanut butter
1 cup dark chocolate chips

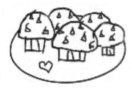

Steps:

1. Preheat the oven to 350°F/175°C.
2. Grease the muffin pan.
3. Combine the dry ingredients in a bowl and then sift them.
4. In another bowl, combine the wet ingredients, then add the dry, sifted ingredients and mix with a spatula. Finally, mix in the chocolate chips.
5. Pour the batter into the muffin pan (each mold should be ¾ of the way full). Bake for 20 to 25 minutes until they are lightly browned and a wooden toothpick will come out clean when you poke them.

CHOCOLATE BROWNIES

Ingredients:

1½ cups cooked and mashed black beans
½ cup agave nectar or pure maple syrup
¼ cup vegetable oil
2 tsp. vanilla
4 Tbsp. cacao powder
½ cup crushed oats
1 tsp. baking powder
½ cup dark chocolate chips

For the frosting:

½ cup dark chocolate chips
1 Tbsp. vegetable oil

Steps:

1. Preheat the oven to 350°F/175°C.
2. Mix the wet ingredients for the brownies in a bowl and then fold in the dry ingredients with a spatula.
3. Stir the chocolate chips into the batter.
4. Grease a square baking pan and pour the brownie batter into it. Bake for 20 to 25 minutes.
5. Remove the pan from the oven and let it cool for 10 minutes.
6. Melt the half cup of chocolate chips with the oil. Pour it over the brownies and let it sit for 15 minutes.
7. Remove the brownies from the pan and cut them in squares.

Note: The brownies should be moist. If you overcook them, they'll dry out. It's important to remove them from the pan—that way, the inner layer will be moist and delicious.

Did you like my book?

It would mean the world if you write a review on Amazon.

Thanks a million!

Ximena

Believe.
Transform.
Be.

INDEX

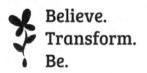 **Believe.**
Transform.
Be.

ABOUT THE AUTHOR

Ximena (pronounced He-men-a) believes in a world that offers opportunities to all its inhabitants and considers our most generous action to deliver a healthy, bountiful planet to future generations. For more than 20 years, she held the position of Chief Financial Officer for Fondo Mexicano para la Conservación de la Naturaleza, a major environmental fund that channels its efforts toward preserving Mexico's beautiful natural resources.

Suffering from long-term and chronic illnesse—and being able to overcome them through nutrition and lifestyle—led Ximena to explore alternatives for personal and professional transformation. She is a certified Level I and II Reiki practitioner and an RYS 200 yoga instructor. She finished her studies as an Integrative Nutrition Health Coach at the Institute for Integrative Nutrition in New York and was one of eight nomination recipients of the Leadership in Health Coaching Award. She was granted as a Certified International Health Coach by the International Association for Health Coaches. She also has a bachelor's degree in public accounting from Instituto Tecnológico Autónomo de México and completed the credits of a master's degree in information technology and business from the same institute.

Ximena founded Believe.Transform.Be to help those who are going through difficult situations to achieve a healthy lifestyle in harmony with the planet through conscious eating. She is dedicated to accompanying her clients during their life transformation processes, to regain their vitality and energy, and offers comprehensive tools that allow them to flourish in all areas of their lives while simultaneously caring for our planet.

Ximena is a sought-after, engaging bi-lingual speaker, fluent in Spanish and English and her clients describe her as someone who is committed, centered, and spiritual—a warm and welcoming person who takes a genuine interest in others.

To invite Ximena to be a speaker at your next event or to learn more about her work, visit www.BelieveTransformBe.com